THE 365-DAY MEDITERRANEAN DIET

COOKBOOK

Easy and Healthy Recipes for Weight Loss
and Living the Mediterranean Lifestyle

Rose Kiser

Table of Content

Introduction

Let me start off by saying I am not a fan of diets. I personally don't know of any 'diet' that doesn't end badly—with you gaining the weight you lost and then some! So, before we move on, I have to clarify one thing: the Mediterranean diet is not a diet in the traditional sense...it is a lifestyle. Now, I know you're probably thinking, "Yeah, that's what all diets claim," and you won't be wholly wrong. But it is my hope that after reading this cookbook, you'll realize that eating the Mediterranean way is not about changing what you put into your body for only a few weeks or months, it is about changing your relationship with food entirely.

Okay, now that I got that out of the way, let me tell you about my love affair with Mediterranean cuisine. I started following this way of eating after my husband had a health scare, and we were forced to rethink our food choices. We used to eat the standard American diet—a 50/50 split of meat and starch washed down by a tall glass of soda, followed by my favorite, store-bought double-layer brownies. Sounds healthy, right? No wonder my husband had a heart attack!

I'm not going to bore you with all the details, but one thing is for sure, the Mediterranean diet with its colorful fruits and veggies, fatty fish, healthy grains, and a good helping of olive oil changed our lives. We've been following this diet for the last four years and have honestly never felt better.

In this cookbook, I want to share with you the health benefits of eating the Mediterranean way, but I also want to make it as easy as possible for you to replace the standard American diet with healthy, nutritious food. There's a reason why doctors all over the world recommend the Mediterranean diet to their patients; you will soon see why! And, after you're completely convinced that this way of eating is the most beneficial option out there, you'll find various delicious recipes to start your journey to a healthier you.

I've made all the recipes included in this cookbook, and they're always a major hit with friends and family. They find it difficult to believe that eating such delectable meals is in any way part of a wholesome eating plan that will heal you from the inside out and prolong your lifespan.

Your whole body will thank you if you make the change!

Chapter 1: Mediterranean Lifestyle Breakdown

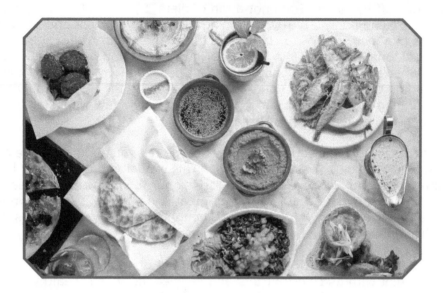

In the 1950s, physiologist Ancel Keys and his colleagues discovered the advantages of following a simple, clean, and wholesome diet (Altomare et al., 2013). They found that the disadvantaged population of Italy had better health than well-off New Yorkers. This was attributed to the fact that fast-food chains were yet to arrive in the Mediterranean Basin.

Keys later went on to lead the Seven Countries Study, where he noticed that there is a link between what you eat, how you live, and cardiovascular disease (Keys et al., 1986). People who followed a Mediterranean diet have a lower risk of developing heart disease and were overall healthier, chiefly due to the high olive oil intake, as well as eating primarily fruits, vegetables, whole grains, beans, and nuts.

The research doesn't stop there. Study after study has shown that the Mediterranean diet is an effective way to prevent cardiovascular disease (Trichopoulou, 2001). And, if you're a woman, there are additional advantages such as warding off chronic diseases linked to old age, including kidney disease, lung disease, and cancer.

What makes the Mediterranean diet so potent is the focus on wholesome, natural foods. The average American diet, on the other hand, involves copious amounts of sugar, refined carbs, saturated fat, and sodium by the spoonful! This leads to obesity, which leads to a slew of other health issues. In fact, 42% of adults in America are obese, and a staggering one in five kids struggle with their weight (Centers for Disease Control and Prevention, 2015).

Those figures alone should convince you to change your eating habits!

In addition to a healthy heart, your brain will stay in tip-top shape well into your golden years when following the Mediterranean diet (American Geriatrics Society, 2017).

It should be apparent why switching from the standard American diet to the Mediterranean will bring nothing but good things your way!

The ABCs of the Mediterranean Diet

Antioxidants, broccoli, chickpeas; you can easily create a plate filled with healthy food starting with each letter of the alphabet! As long as you're eating a balance of high-antioxidant foods, healthy fats, and enough fiber, you're eating the Mediterranean way. Easy, isn't it?

However, as I mentioned in the introduction, the Mediterranean diet is not only about what you fuel your body with; it's about changing your lifestyle. Spending time with your family, exercising, getting enough sleep, and reducing stress all form part of living the Mediterranean way.

I have to mention that the Mediterranean diet does not require you to count calories, weigh your food, or give yourself a headache trying to work out your macronutrients. The only thing you have to do is eat within moderation. That may be difficult if you're trying to lose weight or if you struggle with binge eating, but don't feel dismayed. You will be feeding your body wholesome food, which will make you feel better physically and emotionally, and this will make you instinctively eat less.

But, let's quickly have a look at the foods you'll be enjoying when you follow this diet.

The Mediterranean Food Pyramid

We've all seen the standard food pyramid—carbohydrates and refined grains take up the whole first tier of it! If we pay attention to the research, that's not a good thing at all. Simple carbs—that's your white bread, pasta, cakes, pastries, doughnuts, sweets and candy, soda, everything we Americans love so much—is terrible for you. It plays havoc on your blood sugar and insulin levels, which leads to diabetes and affects your overall well-being negatively (Dyson, 2015).

This is why you'll see a more low-carb approach to the Mediterranean diet in this cookbook. It can only be good for you if you limit your carbohydrate intake to complex carbs like whole grains, oatmeal, etc.

So, let's break down the Mediterranean food pyramid.

Tier one: Reduce stress, get more exercise, spend time with your family, go outside more often—all the lifestyle aspects that will increase the quality of your life.
Tier two: Fruits, veggies, whole grains, beans and legumes, nuts, seeds, herbs and spices, olive oil, and other good fats. It is recommended that you eat these foods daily.

Tier three: Fish, seafood, poultry, eggs, and dairy. You can eat these foods three to five times a week, but poultry, eggs, and dairy portions should be smaller than fish and seafood.

Tier four: Red meat, rice, pasta, potatoes, refined flour products, and sweets. These types of food you should limit as much as possible. I'd say treat yourself to eating it once or twice a month and no more.

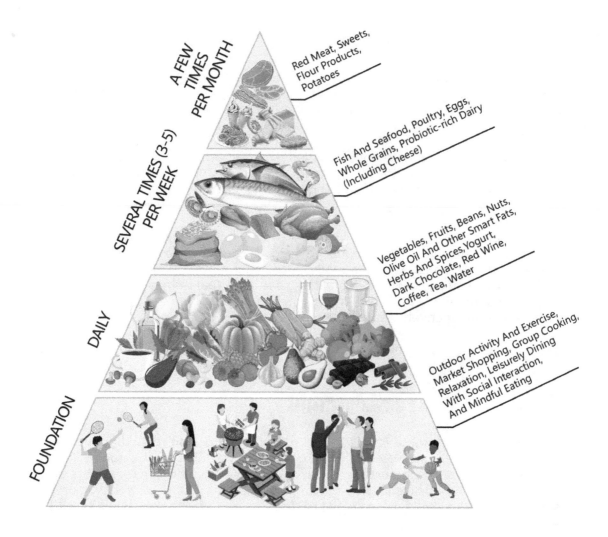

A FEW TIMES PER MONTH
Red Meat, Sweets, Flour Products, Potatoes
SEVERAL TIMES (3-5) PER WEEK
Fish And Seafood, Poultry, Eggs, Whole Grains, Probiotic-rich Dairy (Including Cheese)
DAILY
Vegetables, Fruits, Beans, Nuts, Olive Oil And Other Smart Fats, Herbs And Spices,Yogurt, Dark Chocolate, Red Wine, Coffee, Tea, Water
FOUNDATION
Outdoor Activity And Exercise, Market Shopping, Group Cooking, Relaxation, Leisurely Dining With Social Interaction, And Mindful Eating

Foods to Enjoy

Your plate will, most of the time, be packed to the brim with a colorful array of vegetables since the Mediterranean diet is primarily plant-based.

Let's look at the types of food that are staples in this diet.

Whole grains

Whole grains are superior to refined grains because they haven't been stripped of the fibrous layer that also contains all the vitamins and nutrients. Quinoa, barley, kasha, and oatmeal (I highly recommend steel cut oats for maximum benefit) are some of the healthy grains you'll be consuming with the Mediterranean diet.

Fruits and vegetables

Turn your plate into a rainbow! Colorful vegetables usually contain a lot of phytonutrients and antioxidants that will counter any free radicals. But if you're in the mood to go all-green, that's fine too. The bottom line is that all fruit and veggies are packed with vitamins and minerals and contain a lot of fiber—all of the things you need in your diet.

Nuts

A perfect way to fight hunger pangs in between meals. Nuts contain monounsaturated fat and Omega-3 fatty acids, but they're also a good source of protein. These delicious tiny treats also fight bad cholesterol and promote the overall health of your arteries (Mayo Clinic, n.d.).

Beans and legumes

Beans will make you feel fuller for longer because they are so fiber-rich. Regularly consuming beans will lower your cholesterol and prevent diabetes (Nierenberg, 2014).

Fish

I can't over-emphasize the value of consuming fish on a regular basis. Oily fish like salmon, sardines, trout, herring, flounder, shad, and pollock have a high Omega-3 fatty acid content, which is excellent news. Not getting enough Omega-3 in your diet causes a spike of inflammation in your body that can cause anything from acne to arthritis.

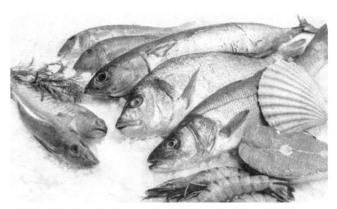

Just keep in mind that fish contain mercury, which is dangerous to pregnant women and children. However, the oilier the fish, the lower its mercury levels, so stick to the fish mentioned above and avoid tilefish, king mackerel, shark, and swordfish.

Olive oil

Olive oil is high in monounsaturated fat, which is great for your heart. On the Mediterranean diet, olive oil will be your go-to fat, and this means your chances of getting diabetes and heart disease will be decreased. Even more exciting is the fact that olive oil can actually help you lose weight since it will make you feel satiated for longer.

Red wine

Red wine contains two power substances called polyphenols and resveratrol that are linked to heart health. This doesn't mean you can drink a bottle a night—the Mediterranean diet is all about moderation. Limit yourself to one or two 5-ounce glasses a day.

Before the coffee and tea lovers get up in arms, I didn't forget about you! You're more than welcome to drink these beverages but also in moderation. Of course, if you drink green tea, forget about limiting your intake at all. That's one drink (after water) that you can't drink enough of—it's just so good for you.

Dark chocolate

Packed with flavanols—a potent antioxidant—dark chocolate is healthy. Again, self-control is important. What do they say? Too much of a good thing is a bad thing. So, keep the moderation principle in mind when you indulge in some dark chocolate. No more than an ounce at a time, a few times each week.

Forbidden Foods

Okay, the word forbidden may be a little too harsh. The only foods that aren't allowed on the Mediterranean diet are those that are harmful to your health. This includes sugary foods like candy, soda, energy drinks, cookies, and overly processed foods, etc. That being said, there are some foods that you should limit.

Fructose: Throughout our lives, we're told that natural sugars like those found in fruits and honey are good for us when, in actual fact, fructose may even be worse than table sugar. Our bodies don't use this type of sugar for energy—it has no need for it at all. So, fructose gets sent straight to the liver, which, as you can imagine, puts a lot of strain on the liver since it has to convert it all into triglycerides. In turn, the triglycerides get stored as fat, and this increases your risk of heart disease, diabetes, and other health issues linked to excessive fat storage.

Milk: Full-cream milk is high in saturated fat. If you drink milk, make sure it is from grass fed cows, which raises the Omega-3 fatty acid count. Keep in mind, milk contains a lot of calories, and it is never a good idea to drink your calories when you're trying to lose or maintain your weight.

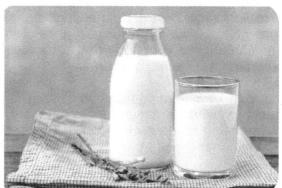

Red meat: Also high in saturated fat, conventional red meat increases your chances of heart disease, hypertension, diabetes, and can cause chronic inflammation when consumed daily. Like milk, and other animal proteins, if you can find beef that is grass-fed, it is higher in Omega-3 fatty acids, so moderate intake can be helpful.

Common Mistakes

Mistakes are unavoidable when you first start the Mediterranean diet—you're changing your relationship with food entirely! I made so many blunders when I started, but at least something good can come from my slip-ups; I can share them with you so that you know what to look out for.

Portion Control
Although you don't have to control your vegetable consumption—since veggies are so fiber-rich, you'll only be able to eat a limited quantity anyway—you do have to keep an eye on everything else on your plate. Nuts and healthy fats are the main culprits because a small amount translates to a lot of calories. This is particularly important if you're following the Mediterranean diet to lose weight.

Carb Overkill
Yes, complex carbs are better for you than refined carbohydrates, but it still doesn't mean you should overindulge. As mentioned earlier, it is better for your health to limit your carb intake—even the right kind of carbs.

Forgetting to Eat Fish

You have to eat enough fish on the Mediterranean diet to reap the heart- and brain-boosting benefits. I know poultry falls on the same tier as fish, but if you have a choice, always choose seafood. You need to get enough of those Omega-3 fatty acids in your diet. If you really struggle to eat enough fish, or you're a vegan, consider fish and seaweed oil supplements.

Consuming the Wrong Dairy

Pasteurized cheese has been stripped of all nutrients and most probiotics. Choose feta, mozzarella, Camembert, or other non-pasteurized cheeses instead to get all the probiotic goodness your gut is craving.

Similarly, artificially flavored yogurt contains a lot of sugar and also doesn't have most probiotics. You can flavor and sweeten plain Greek yogurt with fruits and honey - paying attention to overall sugar and fructose consumption.

As you can see, not all dairy is equal. The more natural option is always better. Sources from grass-fed cows, as mentioned before, should be your go-to.

Limiting the Beans

Beans and legumes are superfoods—so don't leave them off your plate. I know they can take longer to prepare, but they're so excellent at regulating your blood sugar, it's worth the extra effort you have to go through to make them. If you have a pressure cooker, they can be ready within an hour. If necessary, you can also look for canned varieties, but they don't offer the same fiber count and can disrupt blood sugar levels.

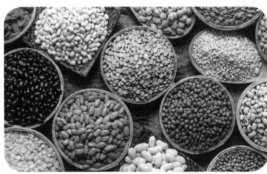

Not Drinking Enough Water

Don't underplay the advantages of drinking enough water. It flushes out toxins from your body, is good for your kidneys and other organs, keeps your digestive system running, and helps keep you satiated; the list of benefits is endless. While we're on the topic of drinking, consuming too much wine is another mistake I made when I started the Mediterranean diet. Remember that you're allowed no more than two 5-ounce glasses of red wine a day.

Overheating Extra-Virgin Olive Oil

Extra-virgin olive oil is best ingested without cooking it. As soon as you heat it and it reaches 400 degrees Fahrenheit, the oil becomes pro-inflammatory. This is damaging to your health. It also tends to lose all its flavor when you overheat it, so it's a waste all-around to cook with extra-virgin olive oil. Reserve it for salad dressing, making your own mayo, or anything else that doesn't require heating. Extra virgin coconut oil is a great option for cooking - although it's a saturated fat, it does have some health benefits, and is also stable at higher temperatures.

You're Not Obeying the 10 Commandments

Yes, the Mediterranean diet comes with its own commandments! I use them as a quick reference if I'm not sure about something since it sums up precisely what the Mediterranean diet is all about.

The ten commandments of the Mediterranean diet and lifestyle are:

❶		Your plate should contain copious amounts of fresh, non-processed foods.
❷		Saturated fat, trans fat, sodium, refined sugar should be banned from your house.
❸		Olive oil is your best friend. Don't cheat on it by using margarine or butter.
❹		Control how much you eat, except when it comes to non-starchy vegetables.
❺		Drink enough water.
❻		Don't drink too much red wine.
❼		Exercise daily.
❽		Don't smoke.
❾		Find ways to relax with your family.
❿		Laugh a lot, smile, and enjoy life.

Eating Out on the Mediterranean Diet

We're social creatures, and that sometimes complicates our lives. It can be extra hard when you're trying to maintain a healthy lifestyle, surrounded by friends and family who don't really care about their health.

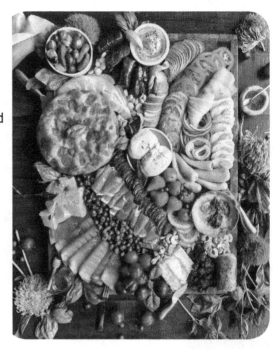

I don't want you to go into a panic when invited out to dinner. I know I used to break out in a light sweat when someone asked me to eat anywhere else other than my own house. But, after I trained myself to spot all the Mediterranean friendly foods, it was a joy to order at restaurants. Of course, being allowed a glass or two of wine with my meal was the cherry on top!

Here are some tips I always use when I dine out with friends or family.

Stick to the Basics

If you know your food pyramid by heart, there is no way that you will order the wrong food. Always choose plant-based dishes over steak with a side of starch; if you can select fish or a seafood dish, even better.

Turn Vegetarian

Vegetarian options on the menu are usually always Mediterranean diet-friendly. They're high in plant-based proteins, contain a lot of fiber and vitamins and nutrients. You'll be eating a well-rounded meal even if you don't have any animal protein on your plate.

Wine Is the Drink of Choice

You're allowed two 5-ounce glasses of wine. I always sip slowly and really enjoy the taste of whatever red I chose. If you're not in the mood for alcohol, you can't go wrong with drinking water. Always stay away from soda—even the diet kind.

Eat Only Half

Portion control isn't something restaurants are known for—unless you're enjoying some French cuisine. I always divide my plate in two if I am worried that I'm overeating. You can take the other half of the food home to eat later.

The Oil Issue

Most restaurants use sunflower and other vegetable oils instead of olive oil—it's cheaper. For this reason, I suggest you avoid any food that is oily. It's always best to select grilled, baked, or roasted. That way, you'll know no harmful oils were used for cooking your food, and you can load up on the olive oil in other ways!

Chapter 2 The 365-Day Mediterranean Diet Program

Diets are diets, when you are forcing yourself into a restricted regimen. However, it would be different if you plant yourself into living the diet, designing your lifestyle around the locus of the diet concept, hence reaping the benefits effortlessly.

Now, this takes 3 baby steps.

◆ First, study the ins and outs of a diet by delving into the introduction, take notes, and make sure you understand the dos and don'ts, what to eat and what to avoid about the diet.

◆ Second, cast out all the unnecessary temptations, make a list of the old habits you are to get rid of, and the new ones to build.

◆ Third, start eating and living the new way, and be patient, give yourself the time to get adapted.

Gradually you will transform into another being, one that would automatically choose the right foods, and living the Mediterranean lifestyle would become your second nature. Notice that time is essential.

Here we have designed a 365-day Mediterranean lifestyle program for you to embark on. We handpick the recipes for you to try daily, and also, we set reminders for you to exercise, to organize a group meal, and to indulge in a moderate cup of your favorite wine. These are the core pillars of a successful Mediterranean lifestyle. In no time, you will find yourself on an easy lane towards success without ever breaking a sweat.

The 365-day Mediterranean lifestyle program can be broken down to 12 months and below we designed the meal plan of the first month, detailing breakfast, lunch, dinner and snack and appetizers, to be more specific, the Mediterranean diet encourages eating plenty of vegetables, grains; moderate fish, and limit red meats to once or twice a month, we have taken this rule into full consideration when designing the meal plan, and also there are essential reminders in the last column of the meal plan chart making sure you are not just minding the food you eat, but also the exercise, the gatherings, the moderate wine... etc. I believe one full month of step-by-step guidance would ease you into the healthy Medi-lifestyle and after one month of implementing this meal plan; you have been Medi-adapted. From this point on, you will be fully capable of recognizing the right food, and making wise diet-decisions, then you can pull up your sleeve and start designing your own Mediterranean meal plan, one that includes your own favorite Mediterranean dishes and serves your own daily routines better.

30-Day Meal Plan Sample

Week 1

Meal Plan	Breakfast	Lunch	Dinner	Snack or Dessert	Reminder
Day-1	Blueberry Smoothie	Fried Eggplant Rolls	Spicy Italian Bean Balls with Marinara	Baby Potato and Olive Salad	
Day-2	Egg Bake	Lush Moroccan Chickpea, Vegetable, and Fruit Stew	Simple Fried Cod Fillets	Ritzy Summer Fruit Salad	
Day-3	Cauliflower Breakfast Porridge	Spicy Tofu Tacos with Cherry Tomato Salsa	Sautéed Green Beans with Tomatoes	Cherry, Plum, Artichoke, and Cheese Board	
Day-4	Morning Overnight Oats with Raspberries	Hearty Butternut Squash, Spinach, and Cheeses Lasagna	Baked Tomatoes and Chickpeas	Root Vegetable Roast	
Day-5	Breakfast Yogurt Sundae	Spicy Grilled Shrimp with Lemon Wedges	Mango and Coconut Frozen Pie	Brown Rice and Black Bean Burgers	
Weekend	Ricotta Toast with Strawberries	Stir-Fry Baby Bok Choy	Slow Cooked Turkey and Brown Rice	Glazed Pears with Hazelnuts	
	Equipped with the recipes in this book, you can organize a group meal or a family dinner and wow them with the newly learned dishes, don't forget to make a toast with your favorite glass of wine and celebrate even tiny achievements you had in aspects of your life. Having a content mindset and enjoying the moment is also key to the Mediterranean diet.				

Week 2

Meal Plan	Breakfast	Lunch	Dinner	Snack or Dessert	Reminder
Day-1	Creamy Peach Smoothie	Ritzy Garden Burgers	Greek Chicken, Tomato, and Olive Salad	Chocolate and Avocado Mousse	
Day-2	Spinach and Egg Breakfast Wraps	Air-Fried Flounder Fillets	Black Bean Chili with Mangoes	Healthy Chia Pudding	
Day-3	Pumpkin Pie Parfait	Sumptuous Vegetable and Cheese Lavash Pizza	Cheesy Peach and Walnut Salad	Pecan and Carrot Cake	
Day-4	Avocado Toast with Goat Cheese	Sardines with Lemony Tomato Sauce	Samosas in Potatoes	Marinated Mushrooms and Olives	
Day-5	Banana-Blueberry Breakfast Cookies	Lentil and Vegetable Curry Stew	Rice and Blueberry Stuffed Sweet Potatoes	Artichoke and Arugula Salad	
Weekend	Easy Buckwheat Porridge	Sweet Pepper Stew	Brown Rice Pilaf with Pistachios and Raisins	Blackberry-Yogurt Green Smoothie	

Equipped with the recipes in this book, you can organize a group meal or a family dinner and wow them with the newly learned dishes, don't forget to make a toast with your favorite glass of wine and celebrate even tiny achievements you had in aspects of your life. Having a content mindset and enjoying the moment is also key to the Mediterranean diet.

Week 3

Meal Plan	Breakfast	Lunch	Dinner	Snack or Dessert	Reminder
Day-1	Mediterranean Eggs (Shakshuka)	Red Pepper Coques with Pine Nuts	Barley, Parsley, and Pea Salad	Apple and Berries Ambrosia	
Day-2	5-Ingredient Quinoa Breakfast Bowls	Greek Vegetable Salad Pita	Baked Lemon Salmon	Raspberry Yogurt Basted Cantaloupe	
Day-3	Creamy Vanilla Oatmeal	Butternut Squash and Cauliflower Coconut Curry Soup	Cheesy Fig Pizzas with Garlic Oil	Lemony Tea and Chia Pudding	
Day-4	Blueberry Smoothie	Mediterranean Braised Cod with Vegetables	Cauliflower Hash with Carrots	Mint Banana Chocolate Sorbet	
Day-5	Cauliflower Breakfast Porridge	Falafel Balls with Tahini Sauce	Italian Sautéd Cannellini Beans	Simple Peanut Butter and Chocolate Balls	
Weekend	Tomato and Egg Scramble	Vegan Lentil Bolognese	Super Cheeses and Mushroom Tart	Simple Spiced Sweet Pecans	

Equipped with the recipes in this book, you can organize a group meal or a family dinner and wow them with the newly learned dishes, don't forget to make a toast with your favorite glass of wine and celebrate even tiny achievements you had in aspects of your life. Having a content mindset and enjoying the moment is also key to the Mediterranean diet.

Week 4

Meal Plan	Breakfast	Lunch	Dinner	Snack or Dessert	Reminder
Day-1	Cheesy Broccoli and Mushroom Egg Casserole	Quinoa and Chickpea Vegetable Bowls with Mango Sauce	Rich Chicken and Small Pasta Broth	Banana, Cranberry, and Oat Bars	
Day-2	Creamy Peach Smoothie	Ritzy Veggie Chili	Cherry, Apricot, and Pecan Brown Rice Bowl	Cucumber Gazpacho	
Day-3	Baked Eggs in Avocado	Lemon-Parsley Swordfish	Mushroom and Soba Noodle Soup	Berry and Rhubarb Cobbler	
Day-4	Breakfast Yogurt Sundae	Glazed Mushroom and Vegetable Fajitas	Grilled Bell Pepper and Anchovy Antipasto	Simple Apple Compote	
Day-5	Crustless Tiropita (Greek Cheese Pie)	Glazed Broiled Salmon	Coconut Blueberries with Brown Rice	Sweet Spiced Pumpkin Pudding	
Weekend	Greens, Fennel, and Pear Soup with Cashews	Baked Rolled Oat with Pears and Pecans	Roasted Tomato Panini	Mini Nuts and Fruits Crumble	

Equipped with the recipes in this book, you can organize a group meal or a family dinner and wow them with the newly learned dishes, don't forget to make a toast with your favorite glass of wine and celebrate even tiny achievements you had in aspects of your life. Having a content mindset and enjoying the moment is also key to the Mediterranean diet.

Ricotta Toast with Strawberries

Prep time: 10 minutes | Cook time: 0 minutes
Serves 2

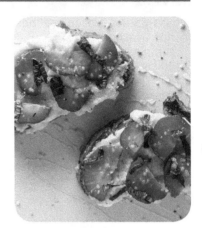

½ cup crumbled ricotta cheese
1 tablespoon honey, plus additional as needed
Pinch of sea salt, plus additional as needed
4 slices of whole-grain bread, toasted
1 cup sliced fresh strawberries
4 large fresh basil leaves, sliced into thin shreds

1. Mix together the cheese, honey, and salt in a small bowl until well incorporated.
2. Taste and add additional salt and honey if needed.
3. Spoon 2 tablespoons of the cheese mixture onto each slice of bread and spread it all over.
4. Sprinkle the sliced strawberry and basil leaves on top before serving.

Tip: If you don't like the honey and cheese, you can omit them. And the strawberries can be replaced with sliced cucumber.

Per Serving
calories: 274 | fat: 7.9g
protein: 15.1g | carbs: 39.8g
fiber: 5.0g | sodium: 322mg

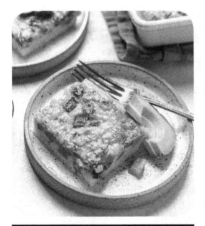

Tips: You can add any of your favorite chopped vegetables to the egg mixture, such as mushrooms, spinach or broccoli. To add more flavors to this meal, serve topped with a sprinkle of shredded cheese.

Per Serving
calories: 240 | fat: 17.4g
protein: 9.0g | carbs: 12.2g
fiber: 2.8g | sodium: 396mg

Egg Bake

Prep time: 10 minutes | Cook time: 30 minutes
Serves 2

1 tablespoon olive oil
1 slice whole-grain bread
4 large eggs
3 tablespoons unsweetened almond milk
½ teaspoon onion powder
¼ teaspoon garlic powder
¾ cup chopped cherry tomatoes
¼ teaspoon salt
Pinch freshly ground black pepper

1. Preheat the oven to 375ºF (190ºC).
2. Coat two ramekins with the olive oil and transfer to a baking sheet. Line the bottom of each ramekin with ½ of bread slice.
3. In a medium bowl, whisk together the eggs, almond milk, onion powder, garlic powder, tomatoes, salt, and pepper until well combined.
4. Pour the mixture evenly into two ramekins. Bake in the preheated oven for 30 minutes, or until the eggs are completely set.
5. Cool for 5 minutes before serving.

Creamy Peach Smoothie

Prep time: 15 minutes | Cook time: 0 minutes
Serves 2

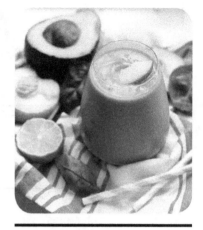

2 cups packed frozen peaches, partially thawed
½ ripe avocado
½ cup plain or vanilla Greek yogurt
2 tablespoons flax meal
1 tablespoon honey
1 teaspoon orange extract
1 teaspoon vanilla extract

1. Place all the ingredients in a blender and blend until completely mixed and smooth.
2. Divide the mixture into two bowls and serve immediately.

Tip: You can serve the smoothie with any toppings of your choice, such as sunflower seeds, chia seeds, cocoa nibs, chopped nuts, or shredded unsweetened coconut.

Per Serving
calories: 212 | fat: 13.1g
protein: 6.0g | carbs: 22.5g
fiber: 7.2g | sodium: 40mg

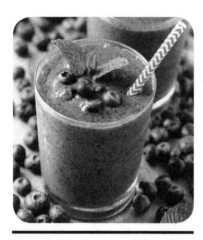

Blueberry Smoothie

Prep time: 5 minutes | Cook time: 0 minutes
Serves 1

1 cup unsweetened almond milk, plus additional as needed
¼ cup frozen blueberries
2 tablespoons unsweetened almond butter
1 tablespoon extra-virgin olive oil
1 tablespoon ground flaxseed or chia seeds
1 to 2 teaspoons maple syrup
½ teaspoon vanilla extract
¼ teaspoon ground cinnamon

1. Blend all the ingredients in a blender until smooth and creamy.
2. You can add additional almond milk to reach your preferred consistency if needed. Serve immediately.

Tip: The blueberries can be replaced with the raspberries or strawberries and the fresh berries will work just as well as frozen in this recipe.

Per Serving
calories: 459 | fat: 40.1g
protein: 8.9g | carbs: 20.0g
fiber: 10.1g | sodium: 147mg

Cauliflower Breakfast Porridge

Prep time: 5 minutes | Cook time: 5 minutes
Serves 2

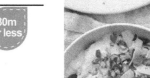

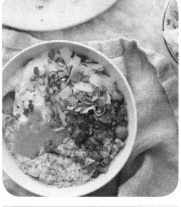

2 cups riced cauliflower
¾ cup unsweetened almond milk
4 tablespoons extra-virgin olive oil, divided
2 teaspoons grated fresh orange peel (from ½ orange)
½ teaspoon almond extract or vanilla extract
½ teaspoon ground cinnamon
⅛ teaspoon salt
4 tablespoons chopped walnuts, divided
1 to 2 teaspoons maple syrup (optional)

1. Place the riced cauliflower, almond milk, 2 tablespoons of olive oil, orange peel, almond extract, cinnamon, and salt in a medium saucepan.
2. Stir to incorporate and bring the mixture to a boil over medium-high heat, stirring often.
3. Remove from the heat and add 2 tablespoons of chopped walnuts and maple syrup (if desired).
4. Stir again and divide the porridge into bowls. To serve, sprinkle each bowl evenly with remaining 2 tablespoons of walnuts and olive oil.

Tip: For a slightly sweeter taste, you can substitute the chopped pecans or shelled pistachios for the walnuts.

Per Serving
calories: 381 | fat: 37.8g
protein: 5.2g | carbs: 10.9g
fiber: 4.0g | sodium: 228mg

Spinach and Egg Breakfast Wraps

Prep time: 10 minutes | Cook time: 7 minutes
Serves 2

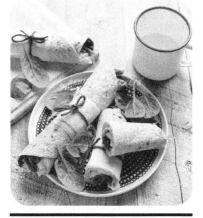

1 tablespoon olive oil
¼ cup minced onion
3 to 4 tablespoons minced sun-dried tomatoes in olive oil and herbs
3 large eggs, whisked
1½ cups packed baby spinach
1 ounce (28 g) crumbled feta cheese
Salt, to taste
2 (8-inch) whole-wheat tortillas

1. Heat the olive oil in a large skillet over medium-high heat.
2. Sauté the onion and tomatoes for about 3 minutes, stirring occasionally, until softened.
3. Reduce the heat to medium. Add the whisked eggs and stir-fry for 1 to 2 minutes.
4. Stir in the baby spinach and scatter with the crumbled feta cheese. Season as needed with salt.
5. Remove the egg mixture from the heat to a plate. Set aside.
6. Working in batches, place 2 tortillas on a microwave-safe dish and microwave for about 20 seconds to make them warm.
7. Spoon half of the egg mixture into each tortilla. Fold them in half and roll up, then serve.

Tip: For a spicy dish, you can use a few teaspoons of harissa sauce to substitute for the sun-dried tomatoes.

Per Serving
calories: 434 | fat: 28.1g
protein: 17.2g | carbs: 30.8g
fiber: 6.0g | sodium: 551mg

Pumpkin Pie Parfait

Prep time: 5 minutes | Cook time: 0 minutes
Serves 4

1 (15-ounce / 425-g) can pure pumpkin purée
4 teaspoons honey
1 teaspoon pumpkin pie spice
¼ teaspoon ground cinnamon
2 cups plain Greek yogurt
1 cup honey granola

1. Combine the pumpkin purée, honey, pumpkin pie spice, and cinnamon in a large bowl and stir to mix well.
2. Cover the bowl with plastic wrap and chill in the refrigerator for at least 2 hours.
3. Make the parfaits: Layer each parfait glass with ¼ cup pumpkin mixture in the bottom. Top with ¼ cup of yogurt and scatter each top with ¼ cup of honey granola. Repeat the layers until the glasses are full.
4. Serve immediately.

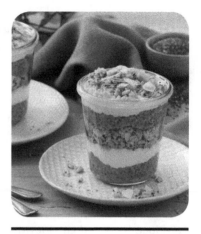

Tip: If you want to make it a gluten-free dish, be sure to use a gluten-free honey granola.

Per Serving
calories: 263 | fat: 8.9g
protein: 15.3g | carbs: 34.6g
fiber: 6.0g | sodium: 91mg

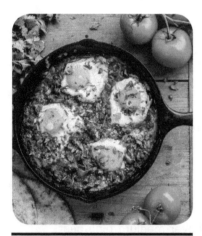

Tip: If you prefer a spicy shakshuka, you can stir in ¼ teaspoon red pepper flakes to the tomatoes.

Per Serving
calories: 223 | fat: 11.8g
protein: 9.1g | carbs: 19.5g
fiber: 3.0g | sodium: 277mg

Mediterranean Eggs (Shakshuka)

Prep time: 5 minutes | Cook time: 20 minutes
Serves 4

30m or less

2 tablespoons extra-virgin olive oil
1 cup chopped shallots
1 teaspoon garlic powder
1 cup finely diced potato
1 cup chopped red bell peppers
1 (14.5-ounce/ 411-g) can diced
tomatoes, drained
¼ teaspoon ground cardamom
¼ teaspoon paprika
¼ teaspoon turmeric
4 large eggs
¼ cup chopped fresh cilantro

1. Preheat the oven to 350ºF (180ºC).
2. Heat the olive oil in an ovenproof skillet over medium-high heat until it shimmers.
3. Add the shallots and sauté for about 3 minutes, stirring occasionally, until fragrant.
4. Fold in the garlic powder, potato, and bell peppers and stir to combine.
5. Cover and cook for 10 minutes, stirring frequently.
6. Add the tomatoes, cardamon, paprika, and turmeric and mix well.
7. When the mixture begins to bubble, remove from the heat and crack the eggs into the skillet.
8. Transfer the skillet to the preheated oven and bake for 5 to 10 minutes, or until the egg whites are set and the yolks are cooked to your liking.
9. Remove from the oven and garnish with the cilantro before serving.

Morning Overnight Oats with Raspberries

Prep time: 5 minutes | Cook time: 0 minutes
Serves 2

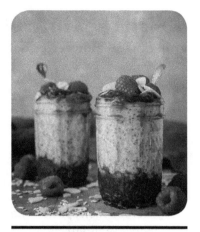

$^2/_3$ cup unsweetened almond milk
¼ cup raspberries
$^1/_3$ cup rolled oats
1 teaspoon honey
¼ teaspoon turmeric
⅛ teaspoon ground cinnamon
Pinch ground cloves

1. Place the almond milk, raspberries, rolled oats, honey, turmeric, cinnamon, and cloves in a mason jar. Cover and shake to combine.
2. Transfer to the refrigerator for at least 8 hours, preferably 24 hours.
3. Serve chilled.

Tip: For added crunch and flavor, you can serve it with any of your favorite toppings, such as chopped nuts, shredded coconut or fruits.

Per Serving
calories: 81 | fat: 1.9g
protein: 2.1g | carbs: 13.8g
fiber: 3.0g | sodium: 97mg

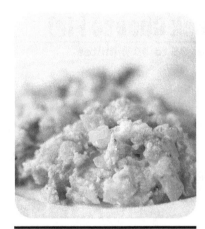

Tips: For an extra dose of micronutrients, try adding sautéed kale or spinach to this tomato and egg scramble. And fresh herbs (1 to 2 teaspoons) will work just as well as dried in this dish.

Per Serving
calories: 260 | fat: 21.9g
protein: 10.2g | carbs: 5.8g
fiber: 1.0g | sodium: 571mg

Tomato and Egg Scramble

Prep time: 10 minutes | Cook time: 20 minutes
Serves 4

30m or less

2 tablespoons extra-virgin olive oil
¼ cup finely minced red onion
1½ cups chopped fresh tomatoes
2 garlic cloves, minced
½ teaspoon dried thyme
½ teaspoon dried oregano
8 large eggs
½ teaspoon salt
¼ teaspoon freshly ground black pepper
¾ cup crumbled feta cheese
¼ cup chopped fresh mint leaves

1. Heat the olive oil in a large skillet over medium heat.
2. Sauté the red onion and tomatoes in the hot skillet for 10 to 12 minutes, or until the tomatoes are softened.
3. Stir in the garlic, thyme, and oregano and sauté for 2 to 4 minutes, or until the garlic is fragrant.
4. Meanwhile, beat the eggs with the salt and pepper in a medium bowl until frothy.
5. Pour the beaten eggs into the skillet and reduce the heat to low. Scramble
6. for 3 to 4 minutes, stirring constantly, or until the eggs are set.
7. Remove from the heat and scatter with the feta cheese and mint. Serve warm.

Baked Eggs in Avocado

Prep time: 5 minutes | Cook time: 10 to 15 minutes
Serves 2

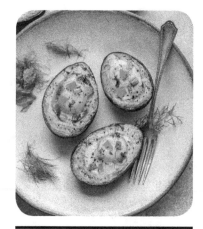

1 ripe large avocado
2 large eggs
Salt and freshly ground black pepper, to taste
4 tablespoons jarred pesto, for serving
2 tablespoons chopped tomato, for serving
2 tablespoons crumbled feta cheese, for serving (optional)

1. Preheat the oven to 425°F (220°C).
2. Slice the avocado in half, remove the pit and scoop out a generous tablespoon of flesh from each half to create a hole big enough to fit an egg.
3. Transfer the avocado halves (cut-side up) to a baking sheet.
4. Crack 1 egg into each avocado half and sprinkle with salt and pepper.
5. Bake in the preheated oven for 10 to 15 minutes, or until the eggs are cooked to your preferred doneness.
6. Remove the avocado halves from the oven. Scatter each avocado half evenly with the jarred pesto, chopped tomato, and crumbled feta cheese (if desired). Serve immediately.

Tip: To add more flavors to this breakfast, you can serve it with your favorite toppings like fresh vegetables or a dollop of plain Greek yogurt.

Per Serving
calories: 301 | fat: 25.9g
protein: 8.1g | carbs: 9.8g
fiber: 5.0g | sodium: 435mg

Crustless Tiropita (Greek Cheese Pie)

Prep time: 10 minutes | Cook time: 35 to 40 minutes
Serves 6

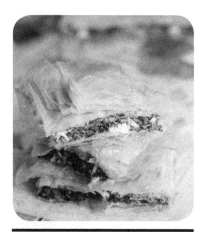

4 tablespoons extra-virgin olive oil, divided
½ cup whole-milk ricotta cheese
1¼ cups crumbled feta cheese
1 tablespoon chopped fresh dill
2 tablespoons chopped fresh mint
½ teaspoon lemon zest
¼ teaspoon freshly ground black pepper
2 large eggs
½ teaspoon baking powder

1. Preheat the oven to 350°F (180°C). Coat the bottom and sides of a baking dish with 2 tablespoons of olive oil. Set aside.
2. Mix together the ricotta and feta cheese in a medium bowl and stir with a fork until well combined. Add the dill, mint, lemon zest, and black pepper and mix well.
3. In a separate bowl, whisk together the eggs and baking powder. Pour the whisked eggs into the bowl of cheese mixture. Blend well.
4. Slowly pour the mixture into the coated baking dish and drizzle with the remaining 2 tablespoons of olive oil.
5. Bake in the preheated oven for about 35 to 40 minutes, or until the pie is browned around the edges and cooked through.
6. Cool for 5 minutes before slicing into wedges.

Tip: To add more flavors to this breakfast, you can serve it with a cup of coffee. It also pairs perfectly with a traditional Greek salad as a light lunch.

Per Serving
calories: 181 | fat: 16.6g
protein: 7.0g | carbs: 1.8g
fiber: 0g | sodium: 321mg

Fluffy Almond Flour Pancakes with Strawberries

Prep time: 5 minutes | Cook time: 15 minutes
Serves 4

1 cup plus 2 tablespoons unsweetened almond milk
1 cup almond flour
2 large eggs, whisked
$1/3$ cup honey
1 teaspoon baking soda
¼ teaspoon salt
2 tablespoons extra-virgin olive oil
1 cup sliced strawberries

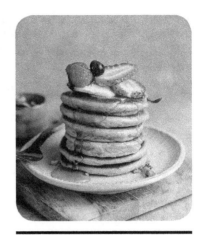

1. Combine the almond milk, almond flour, whisked eggs, honey, baking soda, and salt in a large bowl and whisk to incorporate.
2. Heat the olive oil in a large skillet over medium-high heat.
3. Make the pancakes: Pour $1/3$ cup of batter into the hot skillet and swirl the pan so the batter covers the bottom evenly. Cook for 2 to 3 minutes until the pancake turns golden brown around the edges. Gently flip the pancake with a spatula and cook for 2 to 3 minutes until cooked through. Repeat with the remaining batter.
4. Serve the pancakes with the sliced strawberries on top.

Tip: To add more flavors to this meal, you can serve the pancakes with a drizzle of maple syrup or some fresh fruits like sliced banana or blueberries.

Per Serving
calories: 298 | fat: 11.7g
protein: 11.8g | carbs: 34.8g
fiber: 3.9g | sodium: 195mg

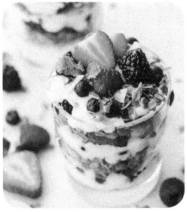

Breakfast Yogurt Sundae

Prep time: 5 minutes | Cook time: 0 minutes
Serves 1

¾ cup plain Greek yogurt
¼ cup fresh mixed berries (blueberries, strawberries, blackberries)
2 tablespoons walnut pieces
1 tablespoon ground flaxseed
2 fresh mint leaves, shredded

1. Pour the yogurt into a tall parfait glass and sprinkle with the mixed berries, walnut pieces, and flaxseed.
2. Garnish with the shredded mint leaves and serve immediately.

Tips: The frozen mixed berries will work just as well as the fresh in this sundae. And you can substitute the cashew or almond pieces for the walnut.

Per Serving
calories: 236 | fat: 10.8g
protein: 21.1g | carbs: 15.9g
fiber: 4.1g | sodium: 63mg

Avocado Toast with Goat Cheese

Prep time: 5 minutes | Cook time: 2 to 3 minutes
Serves 2

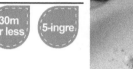

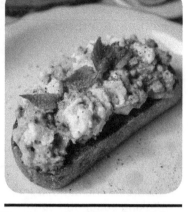

2 slices whole-wheat thin-sliced bread
½ avocado
2 tablespoons crumbled goat cheese
Salt, to taste

1. Toast the bread slices in a toaster for 2 to 3 minutes on each side until browned.
2. Scoop out the flesh from the avocado into a medium bowl and mash it with a fork to desired consistency. Spread the mash onto each piece of toast.
3. Scatter the crumbled goat cheese on top and season as needed with salt.
4. Serve immediately.

Tip: To make this a complete meal, you can serve the avocado toast with any of your favorite toppings, such as crushed nuts, shredded Parmesan cheese, a handful of microgreens, or tomato slices.

Per Serving
calories: 136 | fat: 5.9g
protein: 5.0g | carbs: 17.5g
fiber: 5.1g | sodium: 194mg

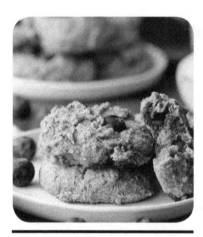

Tip: To make this a complete meal, you can serve it with 1 or 2 hard-boiled eggs.

Per Serving (3 cookies)
calories: 264 | fat: 13.9g
protein: 7.3g | carbs: 27.6g
fiber: 5.2g | sodium: 219mg

Banana-Blueberry Breakfast Cookies

Prep time: 10 minutes | Cook time: 13 minutes
Serves 4

2 medium bananas, sliced
4 tablespoons almond butter
4 large eggs, lightly beaten
½ cup unsweetened applesauce
1 teaspoon vanilla extract
2/3 cup coconut flour
¼ teaspoon salt
1 cup fresh or frozen blueberries

1. Preheat the oven to 375ºF (190ºC). Line a baking sheet with parchment paper.
2. Stir together the bananas and almond butter in a medium bowl until well incorporated.
3. Fold in the beaten eggs, applesauce, and vanilla and blend well.
4. Add the coconut flour and salt and mix well. Add the blueberries and stir to just incorporate.
5. Drop about 2 tablespoons of dough onto the parchment paper-lined baking sheet for each cookie. Using your clean hand, flatten each into a rounded biscuit shape, until it is 1 inch thick.
6. Bake in the preheated oven for about 13 minutes, or until the top is golden brown and a toothpick inserted in the center comes out clean.
7. Let the cookies cool for 5 to 10 minutes before serving.

Blackberry-Yogurt Green Smoothie

Prep time: 5 minutes | Cook time: 0 minutes
Serves 2

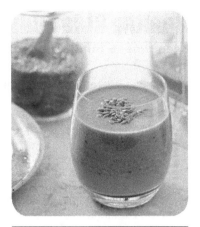

1 cup plain Greek yogurt
1 cup baby spinach
½ cup frozen blackberries
½ cup unsweetened almond milk
½ teaspoon peeled and grated fresh ginger
¼ cup chopped pecans

1. Process the yogurt, baby spinach, blackberries, almond milk, and ginger in a food processor until smoothly blended.
2. Divide the mixture into two bowls and serve topped with the chopped pecans.

Tips: If you prefer a stronger flavor, you can use the fresh turmeric. For extra healthy fats, protein and carbohydrates, you can increase the amount of chopped pecans.

Per Serving
calories: 201 | fat: 14.5g
protein: 7.1g | carbs: 14.9g
fiber: 4.3g | sodium: 103mg

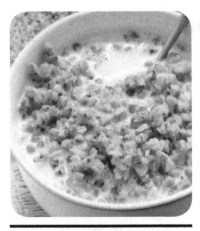

Tip: To add more flavors to this meal, you can serve it with sliced banana, fresh berries, chopped nuts, or a dollop of plain Greek yogurt.

Per Serving
calories: 121 | fat: 1.0g
protein: 6.3g | carbs: 21.5g
fiber: 3.0g | sodium: 47mg

Easy Buckwheat Porridge

Prep time: 5 minutes | Cook time: 40 minutes
Serves 4

3 cups water
2 cups raw buckwheat groats
Pinch sea salt
1 cup unsweetened almond milk

1. In a medium saucepan, add the water, buckwheat groats, and sea salt and bring to a boil over medium-high heat.
2. Once it starts to boil, reduce the heat to low. Cook for about 20 minutes, stirring occasionally, or until most of the water is absorbed.
3. Fold in the almond milk and whisk well. Continue cooking for about 15 minutes, or until the buckwheat groats are very softened.
4. Ladle the porridge into bowls and serve warm.

Healthy Chia Pudding

Prep time: 5 minutes | Cook time: 0 minutes
Serves 4

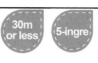
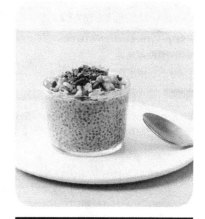

4 cups unsweetened almond milk
¾ cup chia seeds
1 teaspoon ground cinnamon
Pinch sea salt

1. In a medium bowl, whisk together the almond milk, chia seeds, cinnamon, and sea salt until well incorporated.
2. Cover and transfer to the refrigerator to thicken for about 1 hour, or until a pudding-like texture is achieved.
3. Serve chilled.

Tip: You can serve it with your favorite toppings, like blueberries or raspberries. This chia pudding is the perfect healthy breakfast or snack to meal prep.

Per Serving
calories: 236 | fat: 9.8g
protein: 13.1g | carbs: 24.8g
fiber: 11.0g | sodium: 133mg

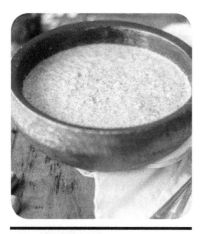

Tip: For added crunch and flavor, sprinkle the fresh berries, chopped peaches, sliced almonds, sunflower seeds, or flaxseeds on top before serving.

Per Serving
calories: 117 | fat: 2.2g
protein: 4.3g | carbs: 20.0g
fiber: 3.8g | sodium: 38mg

Creamy Vanilla Oatmeal

Prep time: 5 minutes | Cook time: 40 minutes
Serves 4

4 cups water
Pinch sea salt
1 cup steel-cut oats
¾ cup unsweetened almond milk
2 teaspoons pure vanilla extract

1. Add the water and salt to a large saucepan over high heat and bring to a boil.
2. Once boiling, reduce the heat to low and add the oats. Mix well and cook for 30 minutes, stirring occasionally.
3. Fold in the almond milk and vanilla and whisk to combine. Continue cooking for about 10 minutes, or until the oats are thick and creamy.
4. Ladle the oatmeal into bowls and serve warm.

Cheesy Broccoli and Mushroom Egg Casserole

Prep time: 10 minutes | Cook time: 40 minutes
Serves 4

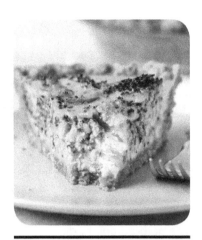

2 tablespoons extra-virgin olive oil
½ sweet onion, chopped
1 teaspoon minced garlic
1 cup sliced button mushrooms
1 cup chopped broccoli

8 large eggs
¼ cup unsweetened almond milk
1 tablespoon chopped fresh basil
1 cup shredded Cheddar cheese
Sea salt and freshly ground black pepper, to taste

1. Preheat the oven to 375ºF (190ºC).
2. Heat the olive oil in a large ovenproof skillet over medium-high heat.
3. Add the onion, garlic, and mushrooms to the skillet and sauté for about 5 minutes, stirring occasionally.
4. Stir in the broccoli and sauté for 5 minutes until the vegetables start to soften.
5. Meanwhile, beat the eggs with the almond milk and basil in a small bowl until well mixed.
6. Remove the skillet from the heat and pour the egg mixture over the top. Scatter the Cheddar cheese all over.
7. Bake uncovered in the preheated oven for about 30 minutes, or until the top of the casserole is golden brown and a fork inserted in the center comes out clean.
8. Remove from the oven and sprinkle with the sea salt and pepper. Serve hot.

Tip: To add more flavors to this meal, you can try adding a can (14.5-ounce / 411-g) of diced tomatoes to this casserole.

Per Serving
calories: 326 | fat: 27.2g
protein: 14.1g | carbs: 6.7g
fiber: 0.7g | sodium: 246mg

5-Ingredient Quinoa Breakfast Bowls

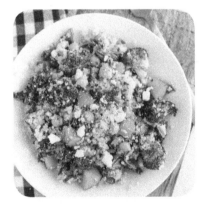

Prep time: 5 minutes | Cook time: 17 minutes
Serves 1

¼ cup quinoa, rinsed
¾ cup water, plus additional as needed
1 carrot, grated
½ small broccoli head, finely chopped
¼ teaspoon salt
1 tablespoon chopped fresh dill

1. Add the quinoa and water to a small pot over high heat and bring to a boil.
2. Once boiling, reduce the heat to low. Cover and cook for 5 minutes, stirring occasionally.
3. Stir in the carrot, broccoli, and salt and continue cooking for 1o to 12 minutes, or until the quinoa is cooked though and the vegetables are fork-tender. If the mixture gets too thick, you can add additional water as needed.
4. Add the dill and serve warm.

Tips: You can try this recipe with different gluten-free grains, such as millet, rolled oats, buckwheat, or sorghum for variety. And you can grind the gluten-free grains in a food processor until they are ground into a powder-like consistency.

Per Serving
calories: 219 | fat: 2.9g
protein: 10.0g | carbs: 40.8g
fiber: 7.1g | sodium: 666mg

Barley, Parsley, and Pea Salad

**Prep time: 10 minutes | Cook time: 10 minutes
Serves 4**

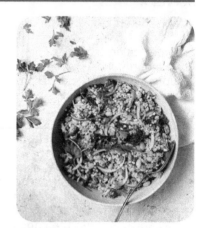

2 cups water
1 cup quick-cooking barley
1 small bunch flat-leaf parsley, chopped (about 1 to 1½ cups)
2 cups sugar snap pea pods
Juice of 1 lemon
½ small red onion, diced
2 tablespoons extra-virgin olive oil
Sea salt and freshly ground pepper, to taste

1. Pour the water in a saucepan. Bring to a boil. Add the barley to the saucepan, then put the lid on.
2. Reduce the heat to low. Simmer the barley for 10 minutes or until the liquid is absorbed, then let sit for 5 minutes.
3. Open the lid, then transfer the barley in a colander and rinse under cold running water.
4. Pour the barley in a large salad bowl and add the remaining ingredients. Toss to combine well.
5. Serve immediately.

Tip: If you have enough time, you can use pearl barley to replace the quick-cooking barley, and it may cost 15 more minutes to simmer the barley.

Per Serving
calories: 152 | fat: 7.4g
protein: 3.7g | carbs: 19.3g
fiber: 4.7g| sodium: 20mg

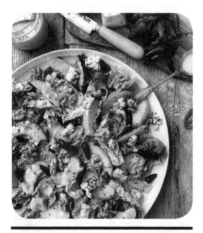

Tip: You can serve this salad as breakfast, and serve it with plain almond yogurt and toss with cubed whole wheat bread, if desired.

Per Serving
calories: 373 | fat: 26.4g
protein: 12.9g | carbs: 27.0g
fiber: 4.7g | sodium: 453mg

Cheesy Peach and Walnut Salad

**Prep time: 10 minutes | Cook time: 0 minutes
Serves 1**

1 ripe peach, pitted and sliced
¼ cup chopped walnuts, toasted
¼ cup shredded Parmesan cheese
1 teaspoon raw honey
Zest of 1 lemon
1 tablespoon chopped fresh mint

1. Combine the peach, walnut, and cheese in a medium bowl, then drizzle with honey. Spread the lemon zest and mint on top. Toss to combine everything well.
2. Serve immediately.

Artichoke and Arugula Salad

Prep time: 10 minutes | Cook time: 0 minutes
Serves 6

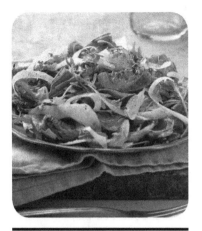

Salad:
6 canned oil-packed artichoke hearts, sliced
6 cups baby arugula leaves
6 fresh olives, pitted and chopped
1 cup cherry tomatoes, sliced in half

Dressing:
1 teaspoon Dijon mustard
2 tablespoons balsamic vinegar
1 clove garlic, minced
2 tablespoons extra-virgin olive oil

For Garnish:
4 fresh basil leaves, thinly sliced

1. Combine the ingredients for the salad in a large salad bowl, then toss to combine well.
2. Combine the ingredients for the dressing in a small bowl, then stir to mix well.
3. Dressing the salad, then serve with basil leaves on top.

Tip: If you don't like canned food, and good at dealing with or want to deal with the fresh artichokes, you can use the same amount of fresh artichoke to replace the canned artichoke hearts.

Per Serving
calories: 134 | fat: 12.1g
protein: 1.6g | carbs: 6.2g
fiber: 3.0g| sodium: 65mg

Baby Potato and Olive Salad

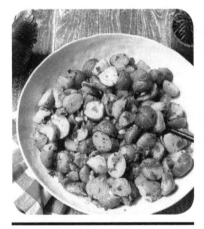

Prep time: 10 minutes | Cook time: 20 minutes
Serves 6

2 pounds (907 g) baby potatoes, cut into 1-inch cubes
1 tablespoon low-sodium olive brine
3 tablespoons freshly squeezed lemon juice (from about 1 medium lemon)
¼ teaspoon kosher salt
3 tablespoons extra-virgin olive oil
½ cup sliced olives
2 tablespoons torn fresh mint
1 cup sliced celery (about 2 stalks)
2 tablespoons chopped fresh oregano

Tip: You can toss the hot tomatoes with half of the olive brine mixture after patting dry and let it to infuse before combining with remaining ingredients.

1. Put the tomatoes in a saucepan, then pour in enough water to submerge the tomatoes about 1 inch.
2. Bring to a boil over high heat, then reduce the heat to medium-low. Simmer for 14 minutes or until the potatoes are soft.
3. Meanwhile, combine the olive brine, lemon juice, salt, and olive oil in a small bow. Stir to mix well.
4. Transfer the cooked tomatoes in a colander, then rinse with running cold water. Pat dry with paper towels.
5. Transfer the tomatoes in a large salad bowl, then drizzle with olive brine mixture. Spread with remaining ingredients and toss to combine well.
6. Serve immediately.

Per Serving
calories: 220 | fat: 6.1g
protein: 4.3g | carbs: 39.2g
fiber: 5.0g | sodium: 231mg

Greek Chicken, Tomato, and Olive Salad

Prep time: 10 minutes | Cook time: 0 minutes
Serves 2

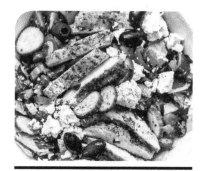

Salad:
2 grilled boneless, skinless chicken breasts, sliced (about 1 cup)

10 cherry tomatoes, halved
8 pitted Kalamata olives, halved
½ cup thinly sliced red onion

Dressing:
¼ cup balsamic vinegar
1 teaspoon freshly squeezed lemon juice
¼ teaspoon sea salt

¼ teaspoon freshly ground black pepper
2 teaspoons extra-virgin olive oil

For Serving:
2 cups roughly chopped romaine lettuce
½ cup crumbled feta cheese

1. Combine the ingredients for the salad in a large bowl. Toss to combine well.
2. Combine the ingredients for the dressing in a small bowl. Stir to mix well.
3. Pour the dressing the bowl of salad, then toss to coat well. Wrap the bowl in plastic and refrigerate for at least 2 hours.
4. Remove the bowl from the refrigerator. Spread the lettuce on a large plate, then top with marinated salad. Scatter the salad with feta cheese and serve immediately.

Tip: How to grill the chicken breast: Preheat the grill to medium high heat, then grease the grill grates with olive oil. Place the chicken breast on the grill grate and grill for 15 minutes or until the internal temperature of the chicken reaches at least 165ºF (74ºC). Flip the chicken breast halfway through. Allow to cool before using.

Per Serving
calories: 328 | fat: 16.9g
protein: 27.6g | carbs: 15.9g
fiber: 3.1g| sodium: 1102mg

Sumptuous Greek Vegetable Salad

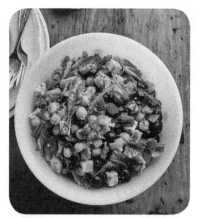

Prep time: 20 minutes | Cook time: 0 minutes
Serves 6

Salad:
1 (15-ounce / 425-g) can chickpeas, drained and rinsed
1 (14-ounce / 397-g) can artichoke hearts, drained and halved
1 head Bibb lettuce, chopped (about 2½ cups)
1 cucumber, peeled deseeded, and chopped (about 1½ cups)
1½ cups grape tomatoes, halved
¼ cup chopped basil leaves
½ cup sliced black olives
½ cup cubed feta cheese

Dressing:
1 tablespoon freshly squeezed lemon juice (from about ½ small lemon)
¼ teaspoon freshly ground black pepper
1 tablespoon chopped fresh oregano
2 tablespoons extra-virgin olive oil
1 tablespoon red wine vinegar
1 teaspoon honey

Tip: You can use ½ head romaine lettuce or other fresh leaves to replace the Bibb lettuce.

Per Serving
calories: 165 | fat: 8.1g
protein: 7.2g | carbs: 17.9g
fiber: 7.0g | sodium: 337mg

1. Combine the ingredients for the salad in a large salad bowl, then toss to combine well.
2. Combine the ingredients for the dressing in a small bowl, then stir to mix well.
3. Dressing the salad and serve immediately.

Roasted Broccoli and Tomato Panzanella

Prep time: 10 minutes | Cook time: 20 minutes
Serves 4

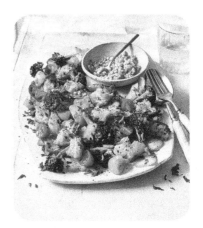

1 pound (454 g) broccoli (about 3 medium stalks), trimmed, cut into 1-inch florets and ½-inch stem slices
2 tablespoons extra-virgin olive oil, divided
1½ cups cherry tomatoes
1½ teaspoons honey, divided
3 cups cubed whole-grain crusty bread
1 tablespoon balsamic vinegar
¼ teaspoon kosher salt
½ teaspoon freshly ground black pepper
¼ cup grated Parmesan cheese, for serving (optional)
¼ cup chopped fresh oregano leaves, for serving (optional)

1. Preheat the oven to 450ºF (235ºC).
2. Toss the broccoli with 1 tablespoon of olive oil in a large bowl to coat well.
3. Arrange the broccoli on a baking sheet, then add the tomatoes to the same bowl and toss with the remaining olive oil. Add 1 teaspoon of honey and toss again to coat well. Transfer the tomatoes on the baking sheet beside the broccoli.
4. Place the baking sheet in the preheated oven and roast for 15 minutes, then add the bread cubes and flip the vegetables. Roast for an additional 3 minutes or until the broccoli is lightly charred and the bread cubes are golden brown.
5. Meanwhile, combine the remaining ingredients, except for the Parmesan and oregano, in a small bowl. Stir to mix well.
6. Transfer the roasted vegetables and bread cubes to the large salad bowl, then dress them and spread with Parmesan and oregano leaves. Toss and serve immediately.

Tip: You can use sun-dried tomatoes, ripped yellow tomatoes, or just grape tomatoes to replace the cherry tomatoes. Remember to reserve the juice and drizzle the salad with the juice for more freshness.

Per Serving
calories: 162 | fat: 6.8g
protein: 8.2g | carbs: 18.9g
fiber: 6.0g | sodium: 397mg

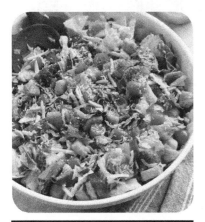

Ritzy Summer Fruit Salad

Prep time: 10 minutes | Cook time: 0 minutes
Serves 8

Salad:
1 cup fresh blueberries
2 cups cubed cantaloupe
2 cups red seedless grapes
1 cup sliced fresh strawberries
2 cups cubed honeydew melon
Zest of 1 large lime
½ cup unsweetened toasted coconut flakes

Dressing:
¼ cup raw honey
Juice of 1 large lime
¼ teaspoon sea salt
½ cup extra-virgin olive oil

1. Combine the ingredients for the salad in a large salad bowl, then toss to combine well.
2. Combine the ingredients for the dressing in a small bowl, then stir to mix well.
3. Dressing the salad and serve immediately.

Tip: You can enjoy this fruit salad between breakfast and lunchtime. Because during this time, the nutritional value of the fruits are highest and they can also give you a bright day.

Per Serving
calories: 242 | fat: 15.5g
protein: 1.3g | carbs: 28.0g
fiber: 2.4g | sodium: 90mg

Brussels Sprout and Apple Slaw

Prep time: 15 minutes | Cook time: 0 minutes
Serves 4

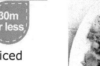

Salad:
1 pound (454 g) Brussels sprouts, stem ends removed and sliced thinly
1 apple, cored and sliced thinly
½ red onion, sliced thinly

Dressing:
1 teaspoon Dijon mustard
2 teaspoons apple cider vinegar
1 tablespoon raw honey
1 cup plain coconut yogurt
1 teaspoon sea salt

For Garnish:
½ cup pomegranate seeds
½ cup chopped toasted hazelnuts

1. Combine the ingredients for the salad in a large salad bowl, then toss to combine well.
2. Combine the ingredients for the dressing in a small bowl, then stir to mix well.
3. Dressing the salad. Let sit for 30 minutes, then serve with pomegranate seeds and toasted hazelnuts on top.

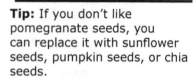

Tip: If you don't like pomegranate seeds, you can replace it with sunflower seeds, pumpkin seeds, or chia seeds.

Per Serving
calories: 248 | fat: 11.2g
protein: 12.7g | carbs: 29.9g
fiber: 8.0g | sodium: 645mg

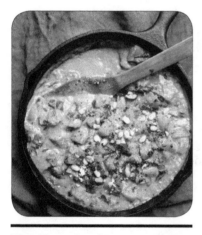

Tip: To make this a complete meal, you can serve this soup with salmon filet or grilled scallops.

Per Serving
calories: 415 | fat: 30.8g
protein: 10.1g | carbs: 29.9g
fiber: 7.0g | sodium: 1386mg

Butternut Squash and Cauliflower Curry Soup

Prep time: 15 minutes | Cook time: 4 hours
Serves 4 to 6

1 pound (454 g) butternut squash, peeled and cut into 1-inch cubes
1 small head cauliflower, cut into 1-inch pieces
1 onion, sliced
2 cups unsweetened coconut milk
1 tablespoon curry powder
½ cup no-added-sugar apple juice
4 cups low-sodium vegetable soup
2 tablespoons coconut oil
1 teaspoon sea salt
¼ teaspoon freshly ground white pepper
¼ cup chopped fresh cilantro, divided

1. Combine all the ingredients, except for the cilantro, in the slow cooker. Stir to mix well.
2. Cook on high heat for 4 hours or until the vegetables are tender.
3. Pour the soup in a food processor, then pulse until creamy and smooth.
4. Pour the puréed soup in a large serving bowl and garnish with cilantro before serving.

Cherry, Plum, Artichoke, and Cheese Board

Prep time: 15 minutes | Cook time: 0 minutes
Serves 4

2 cups rinsed cherries
2 cups rinsed and sliced plums
2 cups rinsed carrots, cut into sticks
1 cup canned low-sodium artichoke hearts, rinsed and drained
1 cup cubed feta cheese

1. Arrange all the ingredients in separated portions on a clean board or a large tray, then serve with spoons, knife, and forks.

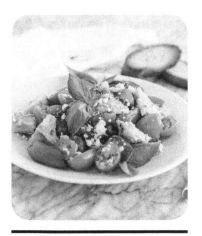

Tip: If you don't like canned food, you can replace the canned artichoke hearts with ½ cup of fresh olives.

Per Serving
calories: 417 | fat: 13.8g
protein: 20.1g | carbs: 56.2g
fiber: 3.0g | sodium: 715mg

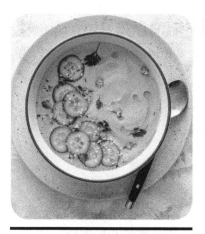

Tip: You can use the almond yogurt or coconut yogurt to replace the plain Greek yogurt, just to make sure they are unsweetened.

Per Serving
calories: 133 | fat: 1.5g
protein: 14.2g | carbs: 16.5g
fiber: 2.9g | sodium: 331mg

Cucumber Gazpacho

Prep time: 10 minutes | Cook time: 0 minutes
Serves 4

2 cucumbers, peeled, deseeded, and cut into chunks
½ cup mint, finely chopped
2 cups plain Greek yogurt
2 garlic cloves, minced
2 cups low-sodium vegetable soup
1 tablespoon no-salt-added tomato paste
3 teaspoons fresh dill
Sea salt and freshly ground pepper, to taste

1. Put the cucumber, mint, yogurt, and garlic in a food processor, then pulse until creamy and smooth.
2. Transfer the puréed mixture in a large serving bowl, then add the vegetable soup, tomato paste, dill, salt, and ground black pepper. Stir to mix well.
3. Keep the soup in the refrigerator for at least 2 hours, then serve chilled.

Hearty Veggie Slaw

Prep time: 20 minutes | Cook time: 0 minutes
Serves 4 to 6

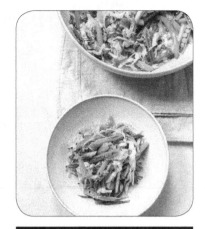

Salad:

2 large broccoli stems, peeled and shredded

½ celery root bulb, peeled and shredded

¼ cup chopped fresh Italian parsley

1 large beet, peeled and shredded

2 carrots, peeled and shredded

1 small red onion, sliced thin

2 zucchinis, shredded

Dressing:

1 teaspoon Dijon mustard

½ cup apple cider vinegar

1 tablespoon raw honey

1 teaspoon sea salt

¼ teaspoon freshly ground black pepper

2 tablespoons extra-virgin olive oil

Topping:

½ cup crumbled feta cheese

1. Combine the ingredients for the salad in a large salad bowl, then toss to combine well.
2. Combine the ingredients for the dressing in a small bowl, then stir to mix well.
3. Dressing the salad, then serve with feta cheese on top.

Tip: You can use this slaw as a side dish to serve with chicken and potato stew or grilled salmon.

Per Serving
calories: 387 | fat: 30.2g
protein: 8.1g | carbs: 25.9g
fiber: 6.0g | sodium: 980mg

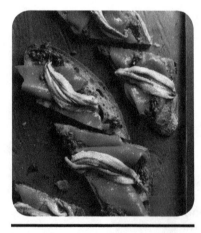

Grilled Bell Pepper and Anchovy Antipasto

Prep time: 15 minutes | Cook time: 8 minutes
Serves 4

2 tablespoons extra-virgin olive oil, divided

4 medium red bell peppers, quartered, stem and seeds removed

6 ounces (170 g) anchovies in oil, chopped

2 tablespoons capers, rinsed and drained

1 cup Kalamata olives, pitted

1 small shallot, chopped

Sea salt and freshly ground pepper, to taste

1. Heat the grill to medium-high heat. Grease the grill grates with 1 tablespoon of olive oil.
2. Arrange the red bell peppers on the preheated grill grates, then grill for 8 minutes or until charred.
3. Turn off the grill and allow the pepper to cool for 10 minutes.
4. Transfer the charred pepper in a colander. Rinse and peel the peppers under running cold water, then pat dry with paper towels.
5. Cut the peppers into chunks and combine with remaining ingredients in a large bowl. Toss to mix well.
6. Serve immediately.

Tip: As an antipasto, you can serve this dish with whole-wheat bread, or you can use it as the filling for whole wheat pita pockets.

Per Serving
calories: 227 | fat: 14.9g
protein: 13.9g | carbs: 9.9g
fiber: 3.8g| sodium: 1913mg

Marinated Mushrooms and Olives

Prep time: 1 hour 10 minutes | Cook time: 0 minutes
Serves 8

1 pound (454 g) white button mushrooms, rinsed and drained
1 pound (454 g) fresh olives
½ tablespoon crushed fennel seeds
1 tablespoon white wine vinegar
2 tablespoons fresh thyme leaves
Pinch chili flakes
Sea salt and freshly ground pepper, to taste
2 tablespoons extra-virgin olive oil

1. Combine all the ingredients in a large bowl. Toss to mix well.
2. Wrap the bowl in plastic and refrigerate for at least 1 hour to marinate.
3. Remove the bowl from the refrigerate and let sit under room temperature for 10 minutes, then serve.

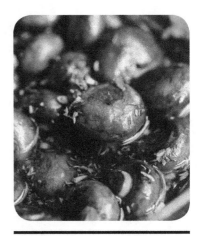

Tip: As a side dish, you can serve it with seared salmon filet or you can pour this dish into a bowl of cooked pasta and stir to serve.

Per Serving
calories: 111 | fat: 9.7g
protein: 2.4g | carbs: 5.9g
fiber: 2.7g | sodium: 449mg

Super Mushroom and Red Wine Soup

Prep time: 40 minutes | Cook time: 35 minutes
Serves 6

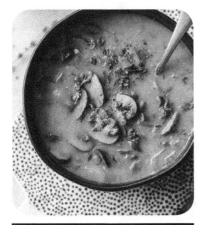

Tip: If you don't have dry red wine, you can use white wine to replace it, such as sherry.

Per Serving
calories: 139 | fat: 7.4g
protein: 7.1g | carbs: 14.4g
fiber: 2.8g | sodium: 94mg

2 ounces (57 g) dried morels
2 ounces (57 g) dried porcini
1 tablespoon extra-virgin olive oil
8 ounces (227 g) button mushrooms, chopped
8 ounces (227 g) portobello mushrooms, chopped
3 shallots, finely chopped
2 cloves garlic, minced
1 teaspoon finely chopped fresh thyme
Sea salt and freshly ground pepper, to taste
1/3 cup dry red wine
4 cups low-sodium chicken broth
½ cup heavy cream
1 small bunch flat-leaf parsley, chopped

1. Put the dried mushrooms in a large bowl and pour in enough water to submerge the mushrooms. Soak for 30 minutes and drain.
2. Heat the olive oil in a stockpot over medium-high heat until shimmering.
3. Add the mushrooms and shallots to the pot and sauté for 10 minutes or until the mushrooms are tender.
4. Add the garlic and sauté for an additional 1 minute or until fragrant. Sprinkle with thyme, salt, and pepper.
5. Pour in the dry red wine and chicken broth. Bring to a boil over high heat.
6. Reduce the heat to low. Simmer for 20 minutes.
7. After simmering, pour half of the soup in a food processor, then pulse until creamy and smooth.
8. Pour the puréed soup back to the pot, then mix in the cream and heat over low heat until heated through.
9. Pour the soup in a large serving bowl and spread with chopped parsley before serving.

Sardines with Lemony Tomato Sauce

Prep time: 10 minutes | Cook time: 40 minutes
Serves 4

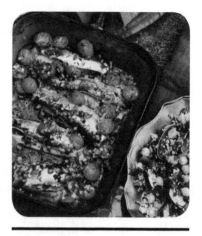

2 tablespoons olive oil, divided
4 Roma tomatoes, peeled and chopped, reserve the juice
1 small onion, sliced thinly
Zest of 1 orange
Sea salt and freshly ground pepper, to taste
1 pound (454 g) fresh sardines, rinsed, spine removed, butterflied
½ cup white wine
2 tablespoons whole-wheat breadcrumbs

1. Preheat the oven to 425ºF (220ºC). Grease a baking dish with 1 tablespoon of olive oil.
2. Heath the remaining olive oil in a nonstick skillet over medium-low heat until shimmering.
3. Add the tomatoes with juice, onion, orange zest, salt, and ground pepper to the skillet and simmer for 20 minutes or until it thickens.
4. Pour half of the mixture on the bottom of the baking dish, then top with the butterflied sardines. Pour the remaining mixture and white wine over the sardines.
5. Spread the breadcrumbs on top, then place the baking dish in the preheated oven. Bake for 20 minutes or until the fish is opaque.
6. Remove the baking sheet from the oven and serve the sardines warm.

Tip: You can replace the whole wheat breadcrumbs with Parmesan cheese shreds to gift the sardines a cheese flavor.

Per Serving
calories: 363 | fat: 20.2g
protein: 29.7g | carbs: 9.7g
fiber: 2.0g| sodium: 381mg

Greens, Fennel, and Pear Soup with Cashews

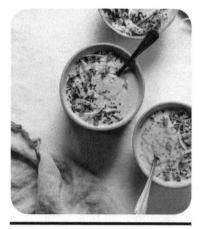

Prep time: 15 minutes | Cook time: 15 minutes
Serves 4 to 6

2 tablespoons olive oil
1 fennel bulb, cut into ¼-inch-thick slices
2 leeks, white part only, sliced
2 pears, peeled, cored, and cut into ½-inch cubes
1 teaspoon sea salt
¼ teaspoon freshly ground black pepper
½ cup cashews
2 cups packed blanched spinach
3 cups low-sodium vegetable soup

1. Heat the olive oil in a stockpot over high heat until shimmering.
2. Add the fennel and leeks, then sauté for 5 minutes or until tender.
3. Add the pears and sprinkle with salt and pepper, then sauté for another 3 minutes or until the pears are soft.
4. Add the cashews, spinach, and vegetable soup. Bring to a boil. Reduce the heat to low. Cover and simmer for 5 minutes.
5. Pour the soup in a food processor, then pulse until creamy and smooth.
6. Pour the soup back to the pot and heat over low heat until heated through.
7. Transfer the soup to a large serving bowl and serve immediately.

Tips: If you like, you can use arugula to replace the spinach. And if you don't like cashews, you can replace it with other kinds of nuts, such as walnuts.

Per Serving
calories: 266 | fat: 15.1g
protein: 5.2g | carbs: 32.9g
fiber: 7.0g | sodium: 628mg

Moroccan Lentil, Tomato, and Cauliflower Soup

Prep time: 15 minutes | Cook time: 4 hours
Serves 6

1 cup chopped carrots
1 cup chopped onions
3 cloves garlic, minced
½ teaspoon ground coriander
1 teaspoon ground cumin
1 teaspoon ground turmeric
¼ teaspoon ground cinnamon
¼ teaspoon freshly ground black pepper
1 cup dry lentils
28 ounces (794 g) tomatoes, diced, reserve the juice
1½ cups chopped cauliflower
4 cups low-sodium vegetable soup
1 tablespoon no-salt-added tomato paste
1 teaspoon extra-virgin olive oil
1 cup chopped fresh spinach
¼ cup chopped fresh cilantro
1 tablespoon red wine vinegar (optional)

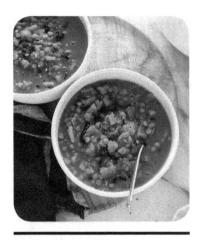

1. Put the carrots and onions in the slow cooker, then sprinkle with minced garlic, coriander, cumin, turmeric, cinnamon, and black pepper. Stir to combine well.
2. Add the lentils, tomatoes, and cauliflower, then pour in the vegetable soup and tomato paste. Drizzle with olive oil. Stir to combine well.
3. Put the slow cooker lid on and cook on high for 4 hours or until the vegetables are tender.
4. In the last 30 minutes during the cooking time, open the lid and stir the soup, then fold in the spinach.
5. Pour the cooked soup in a large serving bowl, then spread with cilantro and drizzle with vinegar. Serve immediately.

Tip: For a healthier choice, you can use the freshly puréed tomato to replace the tomato paste.

Per Serving
calories: 131 | fat: 2.1g
protein: 5.6g | carbs: 25.0g
fiber: 5.5g | sodium: 364mg

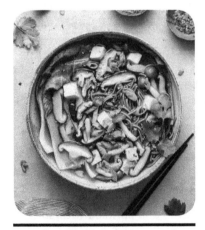

Tip: If you can't find the soda noodles, just use common long pastas to replace it.

Per Serving
calories: 254 | fat: 9.2g
protein: 13.1g | carbs: 33.9g
fiber: 4.0g | sodium: 1773mg

Mushroom and Soba Noodle Soup

Prep time: 15 minutes | Cook time: 10 minutes
Serves 4

2 tablespoons coconut oil
8 ounces (227 g) shiitake mushrooms, stemmed and sliced thin
1 tablespoon minced fresh ginger
4 scallions, sliced thin
1 garlic clove, minced
1 teaspoon sea salt
4 cups low-sodium vegetable broth
3 cups water
4 ounces (113 g) soba noodles
1 bunch spinach, blanched, rinsed and cut into strips
1 tablespoon freshly squeezed lemon juice

1. Heat the coconut oil in a stockpot over medium heat until melted.
2. Add the mushrooms, ginger, scallions, garlic, and salt. Sauté for 5 minutes or until fragrant and the mushrooms are tender.
3. Pour in the vegetable broth and water. Bring to a boil, then add the soba noodles and cook for 5 minutes or until al dente.
4. Turn off the heat and add the spinach and lemon juice. Stir to mix well.
5. Pour the soup in a large bowl and serve immediately.

Pumpkin Soup with Crispy Sage Leaves

Prep time: 15 minutes | Cook time: 10 minutes
Serves 4

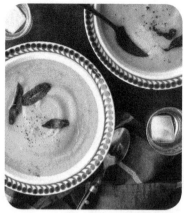

1 tablespoon olive oil
2 garlic cloves, cut into ⅛-inch-thick slices
1 onion, chopped
2 cups freshly puréed pumpkin
4 cups low-sodium vegetable soup
2 teaspoons chipotle powder
1 teaspoon sea salt
½ teaspoon freshly ground black pepper
½ cup vegetable oil
12 sage leaves, stemmed

1. Heat the olive oil in a stockpot over high heat until shimmering.
2. Add the garlic and onion, then sauté for 5 minutes or until the onion is translucent.
3. Pour in the puréed pumpkin and vegetable soup in the pot, then sprinkle with chipotle powder, salt, and ground black pepper. Stir to mix well.
4. Bring to a boil. Reduce the heat to low and simmer for 5 minutes.
5. Meanwhile, heat the vegetable oil in a nonstick skillet over high heat.
6. Add the sage leaf to the skillet and sauté for a minute or until crispy. Transfer the sage on paper towels to soak the excess oil.
7. Gently pour the soup in three serving bowls, then divide the crispy sage leaves in bowls for garnish. Serve immediately.

Tip: You can make your own chipotle powder by combining freshly ground chipotle chiles with garlic powder and herbs you like.

Per Serving
calories: 380 | fat: 20.1g
protein: 8.9g | carbs: 45.2g
fiber: 18.0g | sodium: 1364mg

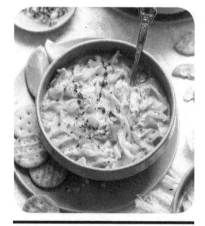

Rich Chicken and Small Pasta Broth

Prep time: 10 minutes | Cook time: 4 hours
Serves 6

6 boneless, skinless chicken thighs
4 stalks celery, cut into ½-inch pieces
4 carrots, cut into 1-inch pieces
1 medium yellow onion, halved
2 garlic cloves, minced
2 bay leaves
Sea salt and freshly ground black pepper, to taste
6 cups low-sodium chicken stock
½ cup stelline pasta
¼ cup chopped fresh flat-leaf parsley

1. Combine the chicken thighs, celery, carrots, onion, and garlic in the slow cooker. Spread with bay leaves and sprinkle with salt and pepper. Toss to mix well.
2. Pour in the chicken stock. Put the lid on and cook on high for 4 hours or until the internal temperature of chicken reaches at least 165ºF (74ºC).
3. In the last 20 minutes of the cooking, remove the chicken from the slow cooker and transfer to a bowl to cool until ready to reserve.
4. Discard the bay leaves and add the pasta to the slow cooker. Put the lid on and cook for 15 minutes or until al dente.
5. Meanwhile, slice the chicken, then put the chicken and parsley in the slow cooker and cook for 5 minutes or until well combined.
6. Pour the soup in a large bowl and serve immediately.

Tip: If you don't have stelline pasta, you can use any other small pastas, such as alphabet pasta.

Per Serving
calories: 285 | fat: 10.8g
protein: 27.4g | carbs: 18.8g
fiber: 2.6g | sodium: 815mg

Roasted Root Vegetable Soup

Prep time: 10 minutes | Cook time: 35 minutes
Serves 6

2 parsnips, peeled and sliced
2 carrots, peeled and sliced
2 sweet potatoes, peeled and sliced
1 teaspoon chopped fresh rosemary
1 teaspoon chopped fresh thyme
1 teaspoon sea salt

½ teaspoon freshly ground black pepper
2 tablespoons extra-virgin olive oil
4 cups low-sodium vegetable soup
½ cup grated Parmesan cheese, for garnish (optional)

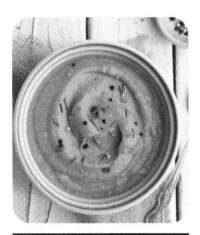

1. Preheat the oven to 400ºF (205ºC). Line a baking sheet with aluminum foil.
2. Combine the parsnips, carrots, and sweet potatoes in a large bowl, then sprinkle with rosemary, thyme, salt, and pepper, and drizzle with olive oil. Toss to coat the vegetables well.
3. Arrange the vegetables on the baking sheet, then roast in the preheated oven for 30 minutes or until lightly browned and soft. Flip the vegetables halfway through the roasting.
4. Pour the roasted vegetables with vegetable broth in a food processor, then pulse until creamy and smooth.
5. Pour the puréed vegetables in a saucepan, then warm over low heat until heated through.
6. Spoon the soup in a large serving bowl, then scatter with Parmesan cheese. Serve immediately.

Tip: If you don't have vegetable soup, just use the same amount of water to replace it.

Per Serving
calories: 192 | fat: 5.7g
protein: 4.8g | carbs: 31.5g
fiber: 5.7g | sodium: 797mg

Root Vegetable Roast

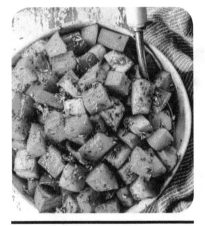

Prep time: 15 minutes | Cook time: 25 minutes
Serves 4 to 6

1 bunch beets, peeled and cut into 1-inch cubes
2 small sweet potatoes, peeled and cut into 1-inch cubes
3 parsnips, peeled and cut into 1-inch rounds
4 carrots, peeled and cut into 1-inch rounds
1 tablespoon raw honey
1 teaspoon sea salt
½ teaspoon freshly ground black pepper
1 tablespoon extra-virgin olive oil
2 tablespoons coconut oil, melted

1. Preheat the oven to 400ºF (205ºC). Line a baking sheet with parchment paper.
2. Combine all the ingredients in a large bowl. Toss to coat the vegetables well.
3. Pour the mixture in the baking sheet, then place the sheet in the preheated oven.
4. Roast for 25 minutes or until the vegetables are lightly browned and soft. Flip the vegetables halfway through the cooking time.
5. Remove the vegetables from the oven and allow to cool before serving.

Tip: If one baking sheet is not large enough to hold all the mixture, then you can use two or more baking sheets to work in batches to avoid overcrowding.

Per Serving
calories: 461 | fat: 18.1g
protein: 5.9g | carbs: 74.2g
fiber: 14.0g | sodium: 759mg

Classic Socca

Prep time: 10 minutes | Cook time: 10 minutes
Serves 4

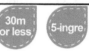
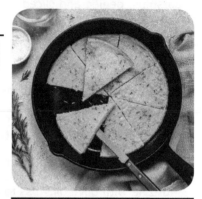

1½ cups chickpea flour
½ teaspoon ground turmeric
½ teaspoon sea salt
½ teaspoon ground black pepper
2 tablespoons plus 2 teaspoons extra-virgin olive oil
1½ cups water

1. Combine the chickpea flour, turmeric, salt, and black pepper in a bowl. Stir to mix well, then gently mix in 2 tablespoons of olive oil and water. Stir to mix until smooth.
2. Heat 2 teaspoons of olive oil in an 8-inch nonstick skillet over medium-high heat until shimmering.
3. Add half cup of the mixture into the skillet and swirl the skillet so the mixture coat the bottom evenly.
4. Cook for 5 minutes or until lightly browned and crispy. Flip the socca halfway through the cooking time. Repeat with the remaining mixture.
5. Slice and serve warm.

Tip: When you cook the second batch of the socca, you can transfer the first batch of cooked socca in a baking pan and keep it warm in the oven under 200ºF (93ºC).

Per Serving
calories: 207 | fat: 10.2g
protein: 7.9g | carbs: 20.7g
fiber: 3.9g | sodium: 315mg

Mashed Grape Tomato Pizzas

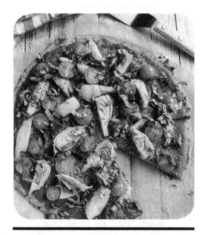

Prep time: 10 minutes | Cook time: 20 minutes
Serves 6

3 cups grape tomatoes, halved
1 teaspoon chopped fresh thyme leaves
2 garlic cloves, minced
¼ teaspoon kosher salt
¼ teaspoon freshly ground black pepper
1 tablespoon extra-virgin olive oil
¾ cup shredded Parmesan cheese
6 whole-wheat pita breads

1. Preheat the oven to 425ºF (220ºC).
2. Combine the tomatoes, thyme, garlic, salt, ground black pepper, and olive oil in a baking pan.
3. Roast in the preheated oven for 20 minutes. Remove the pan from the oven, mash the tomatoes with a spatula and stir to mix well halfway through the cooking time.
4. Meanwhile, divide and spread the cheese over each pita bread, then place the bread in a separate baking pan and roast in the oven for 5 minutes or until golden brown and the cheese melts.
5. Transfer the pita bread onto a large plate, then top with the roasted mashed tomatoes. Serve immediately.

Tip: If you want a more juicy pizza, you can replace the grape tomatoes to normal large tomatoes and chopped the tomatoes into chunks to make them easier for cooking.

Per Serving
calories: 140 | fat: 5.1g
protein: 6.2g | carbs: 16.9g
fiber: 2.0g | sodium: 466mg

Sumptuous Vegetable and Cheese Lavash Pizza

Prep time: 15 minutes | Cook time: 11 minutes
Serves 4

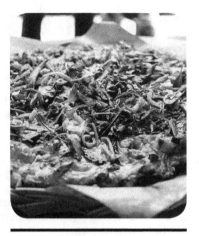

2 (12 by 9-inch) lavash breads
2 tablespoons extra-virgin olive oil
10 ounces (284 g) frozen spinach, thawed and squeezed dry
1 cup shredded fontina cheese
1 tomato, cored and cut into

½-inch pieces
½ cup pitted large green olives, chopped
¼ teaspoon red pepper flakes
3 garlic cloves, minced
¼ teaspoon sea salt
¼ teaspoon ground black pepper
½ cup grated Parmesan cheese

1. Preheat oven to 475ºF (246ºC).
2. Brush the lavash breads with olive oil, then place them on two baking sheet. Heat in the preheated oven for 4 minutes or until lightly browned. Flip the breads halfway through the cooking time.
3. Meanwhile, combine the spinach, fontina cheese, tomato pieces, olives, red pepper flakes, garlic, salt, and black pepper in a large bowl. Stir to mix well.
4. Remove the lavash bread from the oven and sit them on two large plates, spread them with the spinach mixture, then scatter with the Parmesan cheese on top.
5. Bake in the oven for 7 minutes or until the cheese melts and well browned.
6. Slice and serve warm.

Tip: You can replace the tomato, spinach, and olives with broccoli, fennel and artichoke for a different lavash pizza.

Per Serving
calories: 431 | fat: 21.5g
protein: 20.0g | carbs: 38.4g
fiber: 2.5g | sodium: 854mg

Dulse, Avocado, and Tomato Pitas

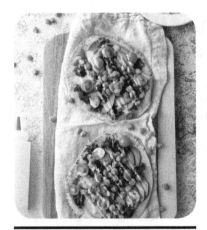

Tip: You can use another lettuce, such as iceberg lettuce, Bibb lettuce, kale, or arugula, to replace the romaine for this recipe.

Per Serving (1 pita)
calories: 412 | fat: 18.7g
protein: 9.1g | carbs: 56.1g
fiber: 12.5g | sodium: 695mg

Prep time: 10 minutes | Cook time: 30 minutes
Makes 4 pitas

2 teaspoons coconut oil
½ cup dulse, picked through and separated
Ground black pepper, to taste
2 avocados, sliced
2 tablespoons lime juice
¼ cup chopped cilantro

2 scallions, white and light green parts, sliced
Sea salt, to taste
4 (8-inch) whole wheat pitas, sliced in half
4 cups chopped romaine
4 plum tomatoes, sliced

1. Heat the coconut oil in a nonstick skillet over medium heat until melted.
2. Add the dulse and sauté for 5 minutes or until crispy. Sprinkle with ground black pepper and turn off the heat. Set aside.
3. Put the avocado, lime juice, cilantro, and scallions in a food processor and sprinkle with salt and ground black pepper. Pulse to combine well until smooth.
4. Toast the pitas in a baking pan in the oven for 1 minute until soft.
5. Transfer the pitas to a clean work surface and open. Spread the avocado mixture over the pitas, then top with dulse, romaine, and tomato slices.
6. Serve immediately.

Greek Vegetable Salad Pita

Prep time: 10 minutes | Cook time: 0 minutes
Serves 4

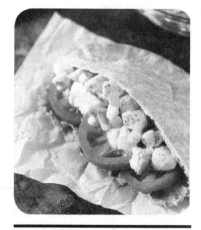

½ cup baby spinach leaves
½ small red onion, thinly sliced
½ small cucumber, deseeded and chopped
1 tomato, chopped
1 cup chopped romaine lettuce
1 tablespoon extra-virgin olive oil
½ tablespoon red wine vinegar
1 teaspoon Dijon mustard
1 tablespoon crumbled feta cheese
Sea salt and freshly ground pepper, to taste
1 whole-wheat pita

1. Combine all the ingredients, except for the pita, in a large bowl. Toss to mix well.
2. Stuff the pita with the salad, then serve immediately.

Tip: If you want to gift your salad pita bread with more flavor, you can sauté the red onion in a nonstick skillet over medium-high heat for 10 minutes or until the onion is caramelized. Stuff the pita with the hot caramelized onion.

Per Serving
calories: 137 | fat: 8.1g
protein: 3.1g | carbs: 14.3g
fiber: 2.4g | sodium: 166mg

Artichoke and Cucumber Hoagies

Prep time: 10 minutes | Cook time: 15 minutes
Makes 1

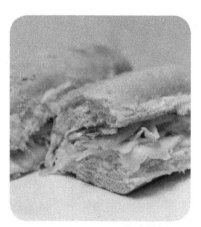

1 (12-ounce / 340-g) whole grain baguette, sliced in half horizontally
1 cup frozen and thawed artichoke hearts, roughly chopped
1 cucumber, sliced
2 tomatoes, sliced
1 red bell pepper, sliced
1/3 cup Kalamata olives, pitted and chopped
¼ small red onion, thinly sliced
Sea salt and ground black pepper, to taste
2 tablespoons pesto
Balsamic vinegar, to taste

1. Arrange the baguette halves on a clean work surface, then cut off the top third from each half. Scoop some insides of the bottom half out and reserve as breadcrumbs.
2. Toast the baguette in a baking pan in the oven for 1 minute to brown lightly.
3. Put the artichokes, cucumber, tomatoes, bell pepper, olives, and onion in a large bowl. Sprinkle with salt and ground black pepper. Toss to combine well.
4. Spread the bottom half of the baguette with the vegetable mixture and drizzle with balsamic vinegar, then smear the cut side of the baguette top with pesto. Assemble the two baguette halves.
5. Wrap the hoagies in parchment paper and let sit for at least an hour before serving.

Tip: You can make your own pesto by combining the minced garlic, crushed pine nuts, dried basil, Parmesan, and salt in a small bowl. Stir to mix well.

Per Serving (1 hoagies)
calories: 1263 | fat: 37.7g
protein: 56.3g | carbs: 180.1g
fiber: 37.8g | sodium: 2137mg

Easy Alfalfa Sprout and Nut Rolls

Prep time: 40 minutes | Cook time: 0 minutes
Makes 16 bite-size pieces

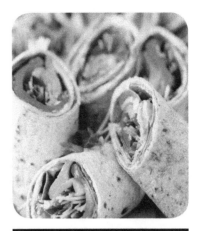

1 cup alfalfa sprouts
2 tablespoons Brazil nuts
½ cup chopped fresh cilantro
2 tablespoons flaked coconut
1 garlic clove, minced
2 tablespoons ground flaxseeds
Zest and juice of 1 lemon
Pinch cayenne pepper
Sea salt and freshly ground black pepper, to taste
1 tablespoon melted coconut oil
2 tablespoons water
2 whole-grain wraps

1. Combine all ingredients, except for the wraps, in a food processor, then pulse to combine well until smooth.
2. Unfold the wraps on a clean work surface, then spread the mixture over the wraps. Roll the wraps up and refrigerate for 30 minutes until set.
3. Remove the rolls from the refrigerator and slice into 16 bite-sized pieces, if desired, and serve.

Tip: You can replace the Brazil nuts with the same amount of almonds, if needed, and put the almonds in a preheated oven to roast over 325ºF (163ºC) for 10 minutes for more flavor.

Per Serving (1 piece)
calories: 67 | fat: 7.1g
protein: 2.2g | carbs: 2.9g
fiber: 1.0g | sodium: 61mg

Mini Pork and Cucumber Lettuce Wraps

Prep time: 20 minutes | Cook time: 0 minutes
Makes 12 wraps

30m or less

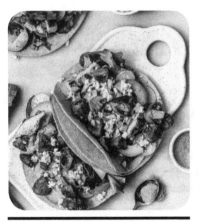

8 ounces (227 g) cooked ground pork
1 cucumber, diced
1 tomato, diced
1 red onion, sliced
1 ounce (28 g) low-fat feta cheese, crumbled
Juice of 1 lemon
1 tablespoon extra-virgin olive oil
Sea salt and freshly ground pepper, to taste
12 small, intact iceberg lettuce leaves

1. Combine the ground pork, cucumber, tomato, and onion in a large bowl, then scatter with feta cheese. Drizzle with lemon juice and olive oil, and sprinkle with salt and pepper. Toss to mix well.
2. Unfold the small lettuce leaves on a large plate or several small plates, then divide and top with the pork mixture.
3. Wrap and serve immediately.

Tip: How to cook the ground pork: Heat 1 tablespoon of olive oil in a nonstick skillet over medium-high heat until shimmering. Add the ground pork and sauté for 5 minutes or until well browned. Remove from the skillet and use immediately.

Per Serving (1 warp)
calories: 78 | fat: 5.6g
protein: 5.5g | carbs: 1.4g
fiber: 0.3g | sodium: 50mg

Samosas in Potatoes

Prep time: 20 minutes | Cook time: 30 minutes
Makes 8

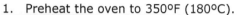

4 small potatoes
1 teaspoon coconut oil
1 small onion, finely chopped
1 small piece ginger, minced
2 garlic cloves, minced
2 to 3 teaspoons curry powder

Sea salt and freshly ground black
pepper, to taste
¼ cup frozen peas, thawed
2 carrots, grated
¼ cup chopped fresh cilantro

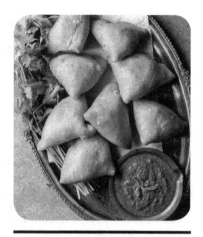

1. Preheat the oven to 350ºF (180ºC).
2. Poke small holes into potatoes with a fork, then wrap with aluminum foil.
3. Bake in the preheated oven for 30 minutes until tender.
4. Meanwhile, heat the coconut oil in a nonstick skillet over medium-high heat until melted.
5. Add the onion and sauté for 5 minutes or until translucent.
6. Add the ginger and garlic to the skillet and sauté for 3 minutes or until fragrant.
7. Add the curry power, salt, and ground black pepper, then stir to coat the onion. Remove them from the heat.
8. When the cooking of potatoes is complete, remove the potatoes from the foil and slice in half.
9. Hollow to potato halves with a spoon, then combine the potato fresh with sautéed onion, peas, carrots, and cilantro in a large bowl. Stir to mix well.
10. Spoon the mixture back to the tomato skins and serve immediately.

Tip: You can replace the cilantro with the same amount of parsley, if necessary.

Per Serving (1 samosa)
calories: 131 | fat: 13.9g
protein: 3.2g | carbs: 8.8g
fiber: 3.0g | sodium: 111mg

Spicy Black Bean and Poblano Dippers

Prep time: 20 minutes | Cook time: 21 minutes
Serves 8

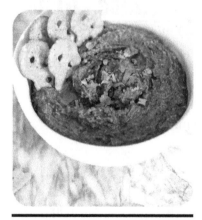

2 tablespoons avocado oil, plus
more for brushing the dippers
1 (15 ounces / 425 g) can black
beans, drained and rinsed
1 poblano, deseeded and
quartered
1 jalapeño, halved and deseeded
½ cup fresh cilantro, leaves and

tender stems
1 yellow onion, quartered
2 garlic cloves
1 teaspoon chili powder
1 teaspoon ground cumin
1 teaspoon sea salt
24 organic corn tortillas

1. Preheat the oven to 400ºF (205ºC). Line a baking sheet with parchment paper and grease with avocado oil.
2. Combine the remaining ingredients, except for the tortillas, in a food processor, then pulse until chopped finely and the mixture holds together. Make sure not to purée the mixture.
3. Warm the tortillas on the baking sheet in the preheated oven for 1 minute or until softened.
4. Add a tablespoon of the mixture in the middle of each tortilla. Fold one side of the tortillas over the mixture and tuck to roll them up tightly to make the dippers.
5. Arrange the dippers on the baking sheet and brush them with avocado oil. Bake in the oven for 20 minutes or until well browned. Flip the dippers halfway through the cooking time.
6. Serve immediately.

Tip: For more flavor, you can serve the dippers with homemade pesto, tomato paste, or other sauce you like.

Per Serving
calories: 388 | fat: 6.5g
protein: 16.2g | carbs: 69.6g
fiber: 13.5g | sodium: 340mg

Roasted Tomato Panini

Prep time: 15 minutes | Cook time: 3 hours 6 minutes
Serves 2

2 teaspoons olive oil
4 Roma tomatoes, halved
4 cloves garlic
1 tablespoon Italian seasoning
Sea salt and freshly ground pepper, to taste
4 slices whole-grain bread
4 basil leaves
2 slices fresh Mozzarella cheese

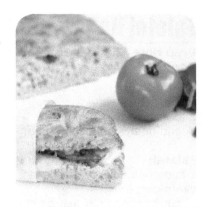

1. Preheat the oven to 250ºF (121ºC). Grease a baking pan with olive oil.
2. Place the tomatoes and garlic in the baking pan, then sprinkle with Italian seasoning, salt, and ground pepper. Toss to coat well.
3. Roast in the preheated oven for 3 hours or until the tomatoes are lightly wilted.
4. Preheat the panini press.
5. Make the panini: Place two slices of bread on a clean work surface, then top them with wilted tomatoes. Sprinkle with basil and spread with Mozzarella cheese. Top them with remaining two slices of bread.
6. Cook the panini for 6 minutes or until lightly browned and the cheese melts. Flip the panini halfway through the cooking.
7. Serve immediately.

Tip: Method to make the panini without panini press: Heat a grill pan over medium-high heat, then put the panini in the pan. Press another grill pan over the panini and cook for 6 minutes. Flip the panini halfway through the cooking time.

Per Serving
calories: 323 | fat: 12.0g
protein: 17.4g | carbs: 37.5g
fiber: 7.5g | sodium: 603mg

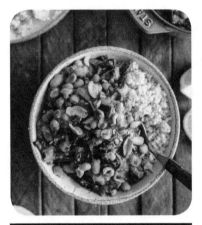

Tip: If you want to remove as much salt that contains in the canned peas as possible, drain the canned peas in a colander and rinse under running cold water, then pat dry with paper towels.

Per Serving
calories: 335 | fat: 16.2g
protein: 12.1g | carbs: 8.3g
fiber: 8.0g | sodium: 214mg

Veg Mix and Blackeye Pea Burritos

Prep time: 15 minutes | Cook time: 40 minutes
Makes 6 burritos

1 teaspoon olive oil
1 red onion, diced
2 garlic cloves, minced
1 zucchini, chopped
1 tomato, diced
1 bell pepper, any color,
deseeded and diced
1 (14-ounce / 397-g) can blackeye peas
2 teaspoons chili powder
Sea salt, to taste
6 whole-grain tortillas

1. Preheat the oven to 325ºF (160ºC).
2. Heat the olive oil in a nonstick skillet over medium heat or until shimmering.
3. Add the onion and sauté for 5 minutes or until translucent.
4. Add the garlic and sauté for 30 seconds or until fragrant.
5. Add the zucchini and sauté for 5 minutes or until tender.
6. Add the tomato and bell pepper and sauté for 2 minutes or until soft.
7. Fold in the black peas and sprinkle them with chili powder and salt. Stir to mix well.
8. Place the tortillas on a clean work surface, then top them with sautéed vegetables mix.
9. Fold one ends of tortillas over the vegetable mix, then tuck and roll them into burritos.
10. Arrange the burritos in a baking dish, seam side down, then pour the juice remains in the skillet over the burritos.
11. Bake in the preheated oven for 25 minutes or until golden brown.
12. Serve immediately.

Falafel Balls with Tahini Sauce

Prep time: 2 hours 20 minutes | Cook time: 20 minutes
Serves 4

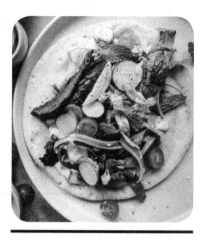

Tahini Sauce:

½ cup tahini
2 tablespoons lemon juice
¼ cup finely chopped flat-leaf
parsley
2 cloves garlic, minced
½ cup cold water, as needed

Falafel:

1 cup dried chickpeas, soaked
overnight, drained
¼ cup chopped flat-leaf parsley
¼ cup chopped cilantro
1 large onion, chopped
1 teaspoon cumin
½ teaspoon chili flakes
4 cloves garlic
1 teaspoon sea salt
5 tablespoons almond flour
1½ teaspoons baking soda,
dissolved in 1 teaspoon water
2 cups peanut oil
1 medium bell pepper, chopped
1 medium tomato, chopped
4 whole-wheat pita breads

Tip: When you fry the falafel balls, if a ball falls apart after you drop it into the oil, then knead more flour into the dough to make it more stable.

Per Serving

calories: 574 | fat: 27.1g
protein: 19.8g | carbs: 69.7g
fiber: 13.4g | sodium: 1246mg

Make the Tahini Sauce:

1. Combine the ingredients for the tahini sauce in a small bowl. Stir to mix well until smooth.
2. Wrap the bowl in plastic and refrigerate until ready to serve.

Make the Falafel:

1. Put the chickpeas, parsley, cilantro, onion, cumin, chili flakes, garlic, and salt in a food processor. Pulse to mix well but not puréed.
2. Add the flour and baking soda to the food processor, then pulse to form a smooth and tight dough.
3. Put the dough in a large bowl and wrap in plastic. Refrigerate for at least 2 hours to let it rise.
4. Divide and shape the dough into walnut-sized small balls.
5. Pour the peanut oil in a large pot and heat over high heat until the temperature of the oil reaches 375ºF (190ºC).
6. Drop 6 balls into the oil each time, and fry for 5 minutes or until golden brown and crispy. Turn the balls with a strainer to make them fried evenly.
7. Transfer the balls on paper towels with the strainer, then drain the oil from the balls.
8. Roast the pita breads in the oven for 5 minutes or until golden brown, if needed, then stuff the pitas with falafel balls and top with bell peppers and tomatoes. Drizzle with tahini sauce and serve immediately.

Glazed Mushroom and Vegetable Fajitas

Prep time: 20 minutes | Cook time: 20 minutes
Makes 6

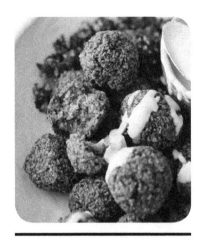

Spicy Glazed Mushrooms:

1 teaspoon olive oil
1 (10- to 12-ounce / 284-
to 340-g) package cremini
mushrooms, rinsed and drained,
cut into thin slices

½ to 1 teaspoon chili powder
Sea salt and freshly ground black
pepper, to taste
1 teaspoon maple syrup

Fajitas:

2 teaspoons olive oil
1 onion, chopped
Sea salt, to taste
1 bell pepper, any color, deseeded
and sliced into long strips
1 zucchini, cut into large

matchsticks
6 whole-grain tortilla
2 carrots, grated
3 to 4 scallions, sliced
½ cup fresh cilantro, finely
chopped

Tip: For more flavor, you can top the fajitas with homemade guacamole or salsa to serve.

Make the Spicy Glazed Mushrooms:

1. Heat the olive oil in a nonstick skillet over medium heat until shimmering.
2. Add the mushrooms and sauté for 10 minutes or until tender.
3. Sprinkle the mushrooms with chili powder, salt, and ground black pepper. Drizzle with maple syrup. Stir to mix well and cook for 5 to 7 minutes or until the mushrooms are glazed. Set aside until ready to use.

Make the Fajitas:

1. Heat the olive oil in the same skillet over medium heat until shimmering.
2. Add the onion and sauté for 5 minutes or until translucent. Sprinkle with salt.
3. Add the bell pepper and zucchini and sauté for 7 minutes or until tender.
4. Meanwhile, toast the tortilla in the oven for 5 minutes or until golden brown.
5. Allow the tortilla to cool for a few minutes until they can be handled, then assemble the tortilla with glazed mushrooms, sautéed vegetables and remaining vegetables to make the fajitas. Serve immediately.

Per Serving

calories: 403 | fat: 14.8g
protein: 11.2g | carbs: 7.9g
fiber: 7.0g | sodium: 230mg

Red Pepper Coques with Pine Nuts

Prep time: 1 day 40 minutes | Cook time: 45 minutes
Makes 4 coques

Dough:
3 cups almond flour
½ teaspoon instant or rapid-rise yeast
2 teaspoons raw honey

1¹/₃ cups ice water
3 tablespoons extra-virgin olive oil
1½ teaspoons sea salt

Red Pepper Topping:
4 tablespoons extra-virgin olive oil, divided
2 cups jarred roasted red peppers, patted dry and sliced thinly
2 large onions, halved and sliced thin

3 garlic cloves, minced
¼ teaspoon red pepper flakes
2 bay leaves
3 tablespoons maple syrup
1½ teaspoons sea salt
3 tablespoons red whine vinegar

For Garnish:
¼ cup pine nuts (optional)
1 tablespoon minced fresh parsley

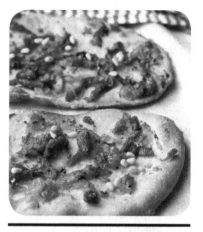

Tip: You can buy four whole-wheat 14 by 5-inch flatbread so you need not make the bread by yourself.

Per Serving (1 coque)
calories: 658 | fat: 23.1g
protein: 3.4g | carbs: 112.0g
fiber: 6.2g | sodium: 1757mg

Make the Dough:
1. Combine the flour, yeast, and honey in a food processor, pulse to combine well. Gently add water while pulsing. Let the dough sit for 10 minutes.
2. Mix the olive oil and salt in the dough and knead the dough until smooth. Wrap in plastic and refrigerate for at least 1 day.

Make the Topping:
1. Heat 1 tablespoon of olive oil in a nonstick skillet over medium heat until shimmering.
2. Add the red peppers, onions, garlic, red pepper flakes, bay leaves, maple syrup, and salt. Sauté for 20 minutes or until the onion is caramelized.
3. Turn off the heat and discard the bay leaves. Remove the onion from the skillet and baste with wine vinegar. Let them sit until ready to use.

Make the Coques:
1. Preheat the oven to 500ºF (260ºC). Grease two baking sheets with 1 tablespoon of olive oil.
2. Divide the dough ball into four balls, then press and shape them into equal-sized oval. Arrange the ovals on the baking sheets and pierce each dough about 12 times.
3. Rub the ovals with 2 tablespoons of olive oil and bake for 7 minutes or until puffed. Flip the ovals halfway through the cooking time.
4. Spread the ovals with the topping and pine nuts, then bake for an additional 15 minutes or until well browned.
5. Remove the coques from the oven and spread with parsley. Allow to cool for 10 minutes before serving.

Spicy Tofu Tacos with Cherry Tomato Salsa

Prep time: 20 minutes | Cook time: 11 minutes
Makes 4 tacos

Cherry Tomato Salsa:
¼ cup sliced cherry tomatoes
½ jalapeño, deseeded and sliced
Juice of 1 lime
1 garlic clove, minced
Sea salt and freshly ground black pepper, to taste
2 teaspoons extra-virgin olive oil

Spicy Tofu Taco Filling:
4 tablespoons water, divided
½ cup canned black beans, rinsed and drained
2 teaspoons fresh chopped chives, divided
¾ teaspoon ground cumin, divided
¾ teaspoon smoked paprika, divided
Dash cayenne pepper (optional)
¼ teaspoon sea salt
¼ teaspoon freshly ground black pepper
1 teaspoon extra-virgin olive oil
6 ounces (170 g) firm tofu, drained, rinsed, and pressed
4 corn tortillas
¼ avocado, sliced
¼ cup fresh cilantro

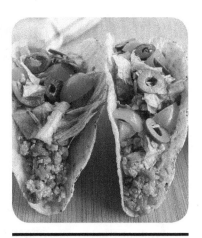

Tip: If you don't like black beans, you can replace it with chickpeas, remember soak the chickpeas in water overnight before using.

Per Serving (1 taco)
calories: 240 | fat: 9.0g
protein: 11.6g | carbs: 31.6g
fiber: 6.7g | sodium: 195mg

Make the Cherry Tomato Salsa:
1. Combine the ingredients for the salsa in a small bowl. Stir to mix well. Set aside until ready to use.

Make the Spicy Tofu Taco Filling:
1. Add 2 tablespoons of water into a saucepan, then add the black beans and sprinkle with 1 teaspoon of chives, ½ teaspoon of cumin, ¼ teaspoon of smoked paprika, and cayenne. Stir to mix well.
2. Cook for 5 minutes over medium heat until heated through, then mash the black beans with the back of a spoon. Turn off the heat and set aside.
3. Add remaining water into a bowl, then add the remaining chives, cumin, and paprika. Sprinkle with cayenne, salt, and black pepper. Stir to mix well. Set aside.
4. Heat the olive oil in a nonstick skillet over medium heat until shimmering.
5. Add the tofu and drizzle with taco sauce, then sauté for 5 minutes or until the seasoning is absorbed. Remove the tofu from the skillet and set aside.
6. Warm the tortillas in the skillet for 1 minutes or until heated through.
7. Transfer the tortillas onto a large plate and top with tofu, mashed black beans, avocado, cilantro, then drizzle the tomato salsa over. Serve immediately.

Mushroom and Caramelized Onion Musakhan

Prep time: 20 minutes | Cook time: 1 hour 5 minutes
Serves 4

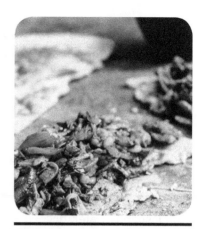

2 tablespoons sumac, plus more for sprinkling
1 teaspoon ground allspice
½ teaspoon ground cardamom
½ teaspoon ground cumin
3 tablespoons extra-virgin olive oil, divided
2 pounds (907 g) portobello mushroom caps, gills removed, caps halved and sliced ½ inch thick
3 medium white onions, coarsely chopped
¼ cup water
Kosher salt, to taste
1 whole-wheat Turkish flatbread
¼ cup pine nuts
1 lemon, wedged

1. Preheat the oven to 350ºF (180ºC).
2. Combine 2 tablespoons of sumac, allspice, cardamom, and cumin in a small bowl. Stir to mix well.
3. Heat 2 tablespoons of olive oil in an oven-proof skillet over medium-high heat until shimmering.
4. Add the mushroom to the skillet and sprinkle with half of sumac mixture. Sauté for 8 minutes or until the mushrooms are tender. You may need to work in batches to avoid overcrowding. Transfer the mushrooms to a plate and set side.
5. Heat 1 tablespoon of olive oil in the skillet over medium-high heat until shimmering.
6. Add the onion and sauté for 20 minutes or until caramelized. Sprinkle with remaining sumac mixture, then cook for 1 more minute.
7. Pour in the water and sprinkle with salt. Bring to a simmer.
8. Turn off the heat and put the mushroom back to the skillet.
9. Place the skillet in the preheated oven and bake for 30 minutes.
10. Remove the skillet from the oven and let the mushroom sit for 10 minutes until cooled down.
11. Heat the Turkish flatbread in a baking dish in the oven for 5 minutes or until warmed through.
12. Arrange the bread on a large plate and top with mushrooms, onions, and roasted pine nuts. Squeeze the lemon wedges over and sprinkle with more sumac. Serve immediately.

Tip: How to roast the pine nuts: Heat 1 tablespoon of olive oil in a separate skillet over medium heat until shimmering. Add the pine nuts and toast for 3 minutes or until lightly browned. Sprinkle with salt and set aside until ready to serve.

Per Serving
calories: 336 | fat: 18.7g
protein: 11.5g | carbs: 34.3g
fiber: 6.9g | sodium: 369mg

Ritzy Garden Burgers

Prep time: 1 hour 30 minutes | Cook time: 30 minutes
Serves 6

1 tablespoon avocado oil
1 yellow onion, diced
½ cup shredded carrots
4 garlic cloves, halved
1 (15 ounces / 425 g) can black beans, rinsed and drained
1 cup gluten-free rolled oats
¼ cup oil-packed sun-dried tomatoes, drained and chopped
½ cup sunflower seeds, toasted

1 teaspoon chili powder
1 teaspoon paprika
1 teaspoon ground cumin
½ cup fresh parsley, stems removed
¼ teaspoon ground red pepper flakes
¾ teaspoon sea salt
¼ teaspoon ground black pepper
¼ cup olive oil

For Serving:
6 whole-wheat buns, split in half and toasted
2 ripe avocados, sliced

1 cup kaiware sprouts or mung bean sprouts
1 ripe tomato, sliced

1. Line a baking sheet with parchment paper.
2. Heat 1 tablespoon of avocado oil in a nonstick skillet over medium heat.
3. Add the onion and carrots and sauté for 10 minutes or until the onion is caramelized.
4. Add the garlic and sauté for 30 seconds or until fragrant.
5. Transfer them into a food processor, then add the remaining ingredients, except for the olive oil. Pulse until chopped fine and the mixture holds together. Make sure not to purée the mixture.
6. Divide and form the mixture into six 4-inch diameter and ½-inch thick patties.
7. Arrange the patties on the baking sheet and wrap the sheet in plastic. Put the baking sheet in the refrigerator and freeze for at least an hour until firm.
8. Remove the baking sheet from the refrigerator, let them sit under room temperature for 10 minutes.
9. Heat the olive oil in a nonstick skillet over medium-high heat until shimmering.
10. Fry the patties in the skillet for 15 minutes or until lightly browned and crispy. Flip the patties halfway through the cooking time. You may need to work in batches to avoid overcrowding.
11. Assemble the buns with patties, avocados, sprouts, and tomato slices to make the burgers.

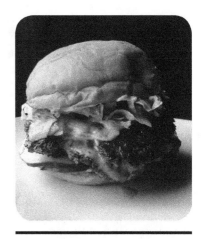

Tip: You can use 6 large romaine lettuce leaves to replace the whole wheat buns to gift your burger with freshness.

Per Serving
calories: 613 | fat: 23.1g
protein: 26.2g | carbs: 88.3g
fiber: 22.9g | sodium: 456mg

Cheesy Fig Pizzas with Garlic Oil

Prep time: 1 day 40 minutes | Cook time: 10 minutes
Makes 2 pizzas

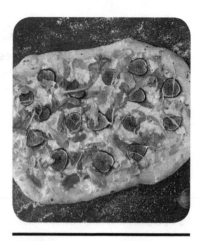

Dough:
1 cup almond flour
1½ cups whole-wheat flour
¾ teaspoon instant or rapid-rise yeast
2 teaspoons raw honey

1¼ cups ice water
2 tablespoons extra-virgin olive oil
1¾ teaspoons sea salt

Garlic Oil:
4 tablespoons extra-virgin olive oil, divided
½ teaspoon dried thyme
2 garlic cloves, minced

⅛ teaspoon sea salt
½ teaspoon freshly ground pepper

Topping:
1 cup fresh basil leaves
1 cup crumbled feta cheese
8 ounces (227 g) fresh figs,

stemmed and quartered lengthwise
2 tablespoons raw honey

Tip: You can replace the garlic oil with homemade pesto and top the pizzas with freshly chopped tomatoes, fried potatoes, and sautéed broccoli.

Per Serving (1 pizza)
calories: 1350 | fat: 46.5g
protein: 27.5g | carbs: 221.9g
fiber: 23.7g | sodium: 2898mg

Make the Dough:
1. Combine the flours, yeast, and honey in a food processor, pulse to combine well. Gently add water while pulsing. Let the dough sit for 10 minutes.
2. Mix the olive oil and salt in the dough and knead the dough until smooth. Wrap in plastic and refrigerate for at least 1 day.

Make the Garlic Oil:
1. Heat 2 tablespoons of olive oil in a nonstick skillet over medium-low heat until shimmering.
2. Add the thyme, garlic, salt, and pepper and sauté for 30 seconds or until fragrant. Set them aside until ready to use.

Make the pizzas:
1. Preheat the oven to 500ºF (260ºC). Grease two baking sheets with 2 tablespoons of olive oil.
2. Divide the dough in half and shape into two balls. Press the balls into 13-inch rounds. Sprinkle the rounds with a tough of flour if they are sticky.
3. Top the rounds with the garlic oil and basil leaves, then arrange the rounds on the baking sheets. Scatter with feta cheese and figs.
4. Put the sheets in the preheated oven and bake for 9 minutes or until lightly browned. Rotate the pizza halfway through.
5. Remove the pizzas from the oven, then discard the bay leaves. Drizzle with honey. Let sit for 5 minutes and serve immediately.

Brown Rice and Black Bean Burgers

Prep time: 20 minutes | Cook time: 40 minutes
Makes 8 burgers

1 cup cooked brown rice
1 (15-ounce / 425-g) can black beans, drained and rinsed
1 tablespoon olive oil
2 tablespoons taco or seasoning
½ yellow onion, finely diced
1 beet, peeled and grated
1 carrot, peeled and grated

2 tablespoons no-salt-added tomato paste
2 tablespoons apple cider vinegar
3 garlic cloves, minced
¼ teaspoon sea salt
Ground black pepper, to taste
8 whole-wheat hamburger buns

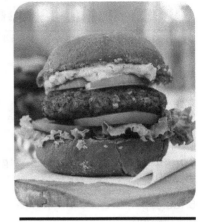

Toppings:
16 lettuce leaves, rinsed well
8 tomato slices, rinsed well

Whole-grain mustard, to taste

1. Line a baking sheet with parchment paper.
2. Put the brown rice and black beans in a food processor and pulse until mix well. Pour the mixture in a large bowl and set aside.
3. Heat the olive oil in a nonstick skillet over medium heat until shimmering.
4. Add the taco seasoning and stir for 1 minute or until fragrant.
5. Add the onion, beet, and carrot and sauté for 5 minutes or until the onion is translucent and beet and carrot are tender.
6. Pour in the tomato paste and vinegar, then add the garlic and cook for 3 minutes or until the sauce is thickened. Sprinkle with salt and ground black pepper.
7. Transfer the vegetable mixture to the bowl of rice mixture, then stir to mix well until smooth.
8. Divide and shape the mixture into 8 patties, then arrange the patties on the baking sheet and refrigerate for at least 1 hour.
9. Preheat the oven to 400ºF (205ºC).
10. Remove the baking sheet from the refrigerator and allow to sit under room temperature for 10 minutes.
11. Bake in the preheated oven for 40 minutes or until golden brown on both sides. Flip the patties halfway through the cooking time.
12. Remove the patties from the oven and allow to cool for 10 minutes.
13. Assemble the buns with patties, lettuce, and tomato slices. Top the filling with mustard and serve immediately.

Tip: How to cook the brown rice: Pour the brown rice in a pot, then pour in enough water to submerge the rice. Bring to a boil over medium-high heat. Reduce the heat to low and simmer for 45 minutes or until most liquid is absorbed and the rice is tender. Remove the rice from the pot and fluff with a fork. Allow to cool for 15 minutes before using.

Per Serving (1 burger)
calories: 544 | fat: 20.0g
protein: 15.8g | carbs: 76.0g
fiber: 10.6g | sodium: 446mg

Turkish Eggplant and Tomatoes Pide with Mint

Prep time: 1 day 40 minutes | Cook time: 20 minutes
Makes 6 pides

Dough:

3 cups almond flour
2 teaspoons raw honey
½ teaspoon instant or rapid-rise yeast

1¹/₃ cups ice water
1 tablespoon extra-virgin olive oil
1½ teaspoons sea salt

Eggplant and Tomato Toppings:

28 ounces (794 g) whole tomatoes, peeled and puréed
5 tablespoons extra-virgin olive oil, divided
1 pound (454 g) eggplant, cut into ½-inch pieces
½ red bell pepper, chopped
Sea salt and ground black

pepper, to taste
3 garlic cloves, minced
¼ teaspoon red pepper flakes
½ teaspoon smoked paprika
6 tablespoons minced fresh mint, divided
1½ cups crumbled feta cheese

Tip: You can buy four whole-wheat 14 by 5-inch flatbread so you need not make the bread by yourself.

Make the Dough:

1. Combine the flour, yeast, and honey in a food processor, pulse to combine well. Gently add water while pulsing. Let the dough sit for 10 minutes.
2. Mix the olive oil and salt in the dough and knead the dough until smooth. Wrap in plastic and refrigerate for at least 1 day.

Make the Toppings:

1. Heat 2 tablespoons of olive oil in a nonstick skillet over medium-high heat until shimmering.
2. Add the bell pepper, eggplant, and ½ teaspoon of salt. Sauté for 6 minutes or until the eggplant is lightly browned.
3. Add the red pepper flakes, paprika, and garlic. Sauté for 1 minute or until fragrant.
4. Pour in the puréed tomatoes. Bring to a simmer, then cook for 10 minutes or until the mixture is thickened into about 3½ cups.
5. Turn off the heat and mix in 4 tablespoons of mint, salt, and ground black pepper. Set them aside until ready to use.

Make the Turkish Pide:

1. Preheat the oven to 500ºF (260ºC). Line three baking sheets with parchment papers.
2. On a clean work surface, divide and shape the dough into six 14 by 5-inch ovals. Transfer the dough to the baking sheets.
3. Brush them with 3 tablespoons of olive oil and spread the eggplant mixture and feta cheese on top.
4. Bake in the preheated oven for 12 minutes or until golden brown. Rotate the pide halfway through the baking time.
5. Remove the pide from the oven and spread with remaining mint and serve immediately.

Per Serving (1 pide)
calories: 500 | fat: 22.1g
protein: 8.0g | carbs: 69.7g
fiber: 5.8g | sodium: 1001mg

Super Cheeses and Mushroom Tart

Prep time: 30 minutes | Cook time: 1 hour 30 minutes
Serves 4 to 6

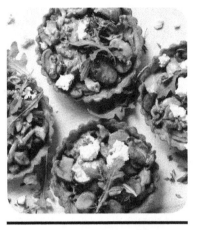

Crust:
1¾ cups almond flour
1 tablespoon raw honey
¾ teaspoon sea salt

¼ cup extra-virgin olive oil
¹/₃ cup water

Filling:
2 tablespoons extra-virgin olive oil, divided
1 pound (454 g) white mushrooms, trimmed and sliced thinly
Sea salt, to taste
1 garlic clove, minced
2 teaspoons minced fresh thyme

¼ cup shredded Mozzarella cheese
½ cup grated Parmesan cheese
4 ounces (113 g) part-skim ricotta cheese
Ground black pepper, to taste
2 tablespoons ground basil

Tip: You can replace the raw honey with the same amount of maple syrup, if needed.

Per Serving
calories: 530 | fat: 26.6g
protein: 11.7g | carbs: 63.5g
fiber: 4.6g | sodium: 785mg

Make the Crust:
1. Preheat the oven to 350ºF (180ºC).
2. Combine the flour, honey, salt and olive oil in a large bowl. Stir to mix well. Gently mix in the water until a smooth dough forms.
3. Drop walnut-size clumps from the dough in the single layer on a tart pan. Press the clumps to coat the bottom of the pan.
4. Bake the crust in the preheated oven for 50 minutes or until firm and browned. Rotate the pan halfway through.

Make the Filling:
1. While baking the crust, heat 1 tablespoon of olive oil in a nonstick skillet over medium-high heat until shimmering.
2. Add the mushrooms and sprinkle with ½ teaspoon of salt. Sauté for 15 minutes or until tender.
3. Add the garlic and thyme and sauté for 30 seconds or until fragrant.

Make the Tart:
1. Meanwhile, combine the cheeses, salt, ground black pepper, and 1 tablespoon of olive oil in a bowl. Stir to mix well.
2. Spread the cheese mixture over the crust, then top with the mushroom mixture.
3. Bake in the oven for 20 minutes or until the cheeses are frothy and the tart is heated through. Rotate the pan halfway through the baking time.
4. Remove the tart from the oven. Allow to cool for at least 10 minutes, then sprinkle with basil. Slice to serve.

Baked Rolled Oat with Pears and Pecans

Prep time: 15 minutes | Cook time: 30 minutes
Serves 6

2 tablespoons coconut oil, melted, plus more for greasing the pan
3 ripe pears, cored and diced
2 cups unsweetened almond milk
1 tablespoon pure vanilla extract
¼ cup pure maple syrup

2 cups gluten-free rolled oats
½ cup raisins
¾ cup chopped pecans
¼ teaspoon ground nutmeg
1 teaspoon ground cinnamon
½ teaspoon ground ginger
¼ teaspoon sea salt

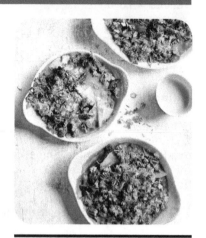

1. Preheat the oven to 350ºF (180ºC). Grease a baking dish with melted coconut oil, then spread the pears in a single layer on the baking dish evenly.
2. Combine the almond milk, vanilla extract, maple syrup, and coconut oil in a bowl. Stir to mix well.
3. Combine the remaining ingredients in a separate large bowl. Stir to mix well. Fold the almond milk mixture in the bowl, then pour the mixture over the pears.
4. Place the baking dish in the preheated oven and bake for 30 minutes or until lightly browned and set.
5. Serve immediately.

Tip: Instead of raisins, you can also use dried berries, apricots, or currants.

Per Serving
calories: 479 | fat: 34.9g
protein: 8.8g | carbs: 50.1g
fiber: 10.8g | sodium: 113mg

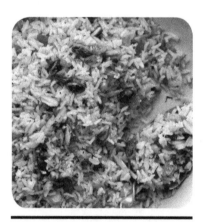

Tip: Instead of using water to cook the brown rice, you can also use unsweetened coconut milk or vegetable soup to increase the nutrition and flavor of the rice.

Per Serving
calories: 264 | fat: 7.1g
protein: 5.2g | carbs: 48.9g
fiber: 4.0g | sodium: 86mg

Brown Rice Pilaf with Pistachios and Raisins

Prep time: 5 minutes | Cook time: 15 minutes
Serves 6

1 tablespoon extra-virgin olive oil
1 cup chopped onion
½ cup shredded carrot
½ teaspoon ground cinnamon
1 teaspoon ground cumin
2 cups brown rice
1¾ cups pure orange juice
¼ cup water
½ cup shelled pistachios
1 cup golden raisins
½ cup chopped fresh chives

1. Heat the olive oil in a saucepan over medium-high heat until shimmering.
2. Add the onion and sauté for 5 minutes or until translucent.
3. Add the carrots, cinnamon, and cumin, then sauté for 1 minutes or until aromatic.
4. Pour int the brown rice, orange juice, and water. Bring to a boil. Reduce the heat to medium-low and simmer for 7 minutes or until the liquid is almost absorbed.
5. Transfer the rice mixture in a large serving bowl, then spread with pistachios, raisins, and chives. Serve immediately.

Italian Sautéd Cannellini Beans

Prep time: 10 minutes | Cook time: 15 minutes
Serves 6

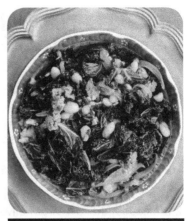

2 teaspoons extra-virgin olive oil
½ cup minced onion
¼ cup red wine vinegar
1 (12-ounce / 340-g) can no-salt-added tomato paste
2 tablespoons raw honey
½ cup water
¼ teaspoon ground cinnamon
2 (15-ounce / 425-g) cans cannellini beans

1. Heat the olive oil in a saucepan over medium heat until shimmering.
2. Add the onion and sauté for 5 minutes or until translucent.
3. Pour in the red wine vinegar, tomato paste, honey, and water. Sprinkle with cinnamon. Stir to mix well.
4. Reduce the heat to low, then pour all the beans into the saucepan. Cook for 10 more minutes. Stir constantly.
5. Serve immediately.

Tip: If you want to remove as much salt that contains in the canned beans as possible, drain the canned beans in a colander and rinse under running cold water, then pat dry with paper towels.

Per Serving
calories: 435 | fat: 2.1g
protein: 26.2g | carbs: 80.3g
fiber: 24.0g | sodium: 72mg

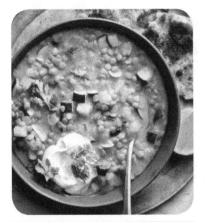

Tip: To make this a complete meal, you can baste it over cooked brown rice.

Per Serving
calories: 530 | fat: 19.2g
protein: 20.3g | carbs: 75.2g
fiber: 15.5g | sodium: 562mg

Lentil and Vegetable Curry Stew

Prep time: 20 minutes | Cook time: 4 hours 7 minutes
Serves 8

1 tablespoon coconut oil
1 yellow onion, diced
¼ cup yellow Thai curry paste
2 cups unsweetened coconut milk
2 cups dry red lentils, rinsed well and drained
3 cups bite-sized cauliflower florets
2 golden potatoes, cut into

chunks
2 carrots, peeled and diced
8 cups low-sodium vegetable soup, divided
1 bunch kale, stems removed and roughly chopped
Sea salt, to taste
½ cup fresh cilantro, chopped
Pinch crushed red pepper flakes

1. Heat the coconut oil in a nonstick skillet over medium-high heat until melted.
2. Add the onion and sauté for 5 minutes or until translucent.
3. Pour in the curry paste and sauté for another 2 minutes, then fold in the coconut milk and stir to combine well. Bring to a simmer and turn off the heat.
4. Put the lentils, cauliflower, potatoes, and carrot in the slow cooker. Pour in 6 cups of vegetable soup and the curry mixture. Stir to combine well.
5. Cover and cook on high for 4 hours or until the lentils and vegetables are soft. Stir periodically.
6. During the last 30 minutes, fold the kale in the slow cooker and pour in the remaining vegetable soup. Sprinkle with salt.
7. Pour the stew in a large serving bowl and spread the cilantro and red pepper flakes on top before serving hot.

Tomato Sauce and Basil Pesto Fettuccine

Prep time: 15 minutes | Cook time: 15 minutes
Serves 4

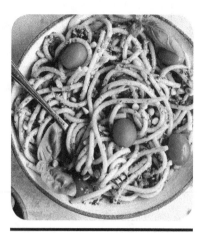

4 Roma tomatoes, diced
2 teaspoons no-salt-added tomato paste
1 tablespoon chopped fresh oregano
2 garlic cloves, minced
1 cup low-sodium vegetable soup
½ teaspoon sea salt
1 packed cup fresh basil leaves
¼ cup pine nuts
¼ cup grated Parmesan cheese
2 tablespoons extra-virgin olive oil
1 pound (454 g) cooked whole-grain fettuccine

1. Put the tomatoes, tomato paste, oregano, garlic, vegetable soup, and salt in a skillet. Stir to mix well.
2. Cook over medium heat for 10 minutes or until lightly thickened.
3. Put the remaining ingredients, except for the fettuccine, in a food processor and pulse to combine until smooth.
4. Pour the puréed basil mixture into the tomato mixture, then add the fettuccine. Cook for a few minutes or until heated through and the fettuccine is well coated.
5. Serve immediately.

Tip: How to cook the fettuccine: Bring a large pot of water to a boil, then add the fettuccine and cook for 8 minutes or until al dente. Drain the fettuccine in a colander before using.

Per Serving
calories: 389 | fat: 22.7g
protein: 9.7g | carbs: 40.2g
fiber: 4.8g | sodium: 616mg

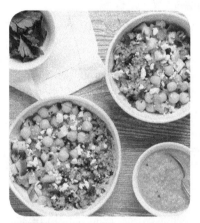

Tip: Instead of maple syrup, you can use the same amount of raw honey for making the mango sauce.

Per Serving
calories: 366 | fat: 11.1g
protein: 15.5g | carbs: 55.6g
fiber: 17.7g | sodium: 746mg

Quinoa and Chickpea Vegetable Bowls

Prep time: 20 minutes | Cook time: 15 minutes
Serves 4

1 cup red dry quinoa, rinsed and drained
2 cups low-sodium vegetable soup
2 cups fresh spinach
2 cups finely shredded red cabbage

1 (15-ounce / 425-g) can chickpeas, drained and rinsed
1 ripe avocado, thinly sliced
1 cup shredded carrots
1 red bell pepper, thinly sliced
4 tablespoons Mango Sauce
½ cup fresh cilantro, chopped

Mango Sauce:
1 mango, diced
¼ cup fresh lime juice
½ teaspoon ground turmeric
1 teaspoon finely minced fresh ginger

¼ teaspoon sea salt
Pinch of ground red pepper
1 teaspoon pure maple syrup
2 tablespoons extra-virgin olive oil

1. Pour the quinoa and vegetable soup in a saucepan. Bring to a boil. Reduce the heat to low. Cover and cook for 15 minutes or until tender. Fluffy with a fork.
2. Meanwhile, combine the ingredients for the mango sauce in a food processor. Pulse until smooth.
3. Divide the quinoa, spinach, and cabbage into 4 serving bowls, then top with chickpeas, avocado, carrots, and bell pepper. Dress them with the mango sauce and spread with cilantro. Serve immediately.

Ritzy Veggie Chili

Prep time: 15 minutes | Cook time: 5 hours
Serves 4

1 (28-ounce / 794-g) can chopped tomatoes, with the juice
1 (15-ounce / 425-g) can black beans, drained and rinsed
1 (15-ounce / 425-g) can red beans, drained and rinsed
1 medium green bell pepper, chopped
1 yellow onion, chopped

1 tablespoon onion powder
1 teaspoon paprika
1 teaspoon cayenne pepper
1 teaspoon garlic powder
½ teaspoon sea salt
½ teaspoon ground black pepper
1 tablespoon olive oil
1 large hass avocado, pitted, peeled, and chopped, for garnish

1. Combine all the ingredients, except for the avocado, in the slow cooker. Stir to mix well.
2. Put the slow cooker lid on and cook on high for 5 hours or until the vegetables are tender and the mixture has a thick consistency.
3. Pour the chili in a large serving bowl. Allow to cool for 30 minutes, then spread with chopped avocado and serve.

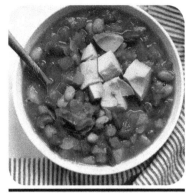

Tip: If you don't like the canned tomatoes, then you can replace them with the same amount of freshly chopped tomatoes and let them sit in a large bowl with their juice.

Per Serving
calories: 633 | fat: 16.3g
protein: 31.7g | carbs: 97.0g
fiber: 28.9g | sodium: 792mg

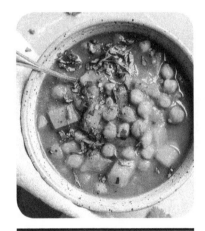

Tip: If you don't like the canned chickpeas, you can use the dried chickpeas and soak them in water overnight before using.

Per Serving
calories: 611 | fat: 9.0g
protein: 30.7g | carbs: 107.4g
fiber: 20.8g | sodium: 344mg

Lush Moroccan Chickpea, Vegetable, and Fruit Stew

Prep time: 20 minutes | Cook time: 6 hours 4 minutes
Serves 6

1 large bell pepper, any color, chopped
6 ounces (170 g) green beans, trimmed and cut into bite-size pieces
3 cups canned chickpeas, rinsed and drained
1 (15-ounce / 425-g) can diced tomatoes, with the juice
1 large carrot, cut into ¼-inch rounds
2 large potatoes, peeled and cubed
1 large yellow onion, chopped
1 teaspoon grated fresh ginger

2 garlic cloves, minced
1¾ cups low-sodium vegetable soup
1 teaspoon ground cumin
1 tablespoon ground coriander
¼ teaspoon ground red pepper flakes
Sea salt and ground black pepper, to taste
8 ounces (227 g) fresh baby spinach
¼ cup diced dried figs
¼ cup diced dried apricots
1 cup plain Greek yogurt

1. Place the bell peppers, green beans, chicken peas, tomatoes and juice, carrot, potatoes, onion, ginger, and garlic in the slow cooker.
2. Pour in the vegetable soup and sprinkle with cumin, coriander, red pepper flakes, salt, and ground black pepper. Stir to mix well.
3. Put the slow cooker lid on and cook on high for 6 hours or until the vegetables are soft. Stir periodically.
4. Open the lid and fold in the spinach, figs, apricots, and yogurt. Stir to mix well.
5. Cook for 4 minutes or until the spinach is wilted. Pour them in a large serving bowl. Allow to cool for at least 20 minutes, then serve warm.

Black Bean Chili with Mangoes

Prep time: 10 minutes | Cook time: 10 minutes
Serves 4

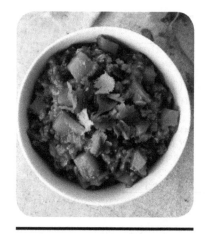

2 tablespoons coconut oil
1 onion, chopped
2 (15-ounce / 425-g) cans black beans, drained and rinsed
1 tablespoon chili powder
1 teaspoon sea salt
¼ teaspoon freshly ground black pepper
1 cup water
2 ripe mangoes, sliced thinly
¼ cup chopped fresh cilantro, divided
¼ cup sliced scallions, divided

1. Heat the coconut oil in a pot over high heat until melted.
2. Put the onion in the pot and sauté for 5 minutes or until translucent.
3. Add the black beans to the pot. Sprinkle with chili powder, salt, and ground black pepper. Pour in the water. Stir to mix well.
4. Bring to a boil. Reduce the heat to low, then simmering for 5 minutes or until the beans are tender.
5. Turn off the heat and mix in the mangoes, then garnish with scallions and cilantro before serving.

Tip: If you don't like to add the sweet taste of mango into the chili, you can replace the mango with avocado chunks, chopped tomatoes, carrots, or potato cubes.

Per Serving
calories: 430 | fat: 9.1g
protein: 20.2g | carbs: 71.9g
fiber: 22.0g | sodium: 608mg

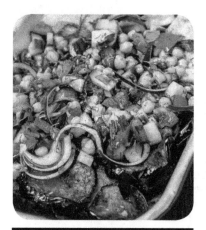

Israeli Style Eggplant and Chickpea Salad

Prep time: 5 minutes | Cook time: 20 minutes
Serves 6

2 tablespoons balsamic vinegar
2 tablespoons freshly squeezed lemon juice
1 teaspoon ground cumin
¼ teaspoon sea salt
2 tablespoons olive oil, divided
1 (1-pound / 454-g) medium globe eggplant, stem removed, cut into flat cubes (about ½ inch thick)

1 (15-ounce / 425-g) can chickpeas, drained and rinsed
¼ cup chopped mint leaves
1 cup sliced sweet onion
1 garlic clove, finely minced
1 tablespoon sesame seeds, toasted

Tip: How to toast the sesame seeds: Before preheating the oven to 550ºF (288ºC), preheat it to 350ºF (180ºC). Pour the sesame seeds in a greased baking dish, then toast in the preheated oven for 8 minutes or until lightly browned and crispy. Stir periodically.

Per Serving
calories: 125 | fat: 2.9g
protein: 5.2g | carbs: 20.9g
fiber: 6.0g | sodium: 222mg

1. Preheat the oven to 550ºF (288ºC) or the highest level of your oven or broiler. Grease a baking sheet with 1 tablespoon of olive oil.
2. Combine the balsamic vinegar, lemon juice, cumin, salt, and 1 tablespoon of olive oil in a small bowl. Stir to mix well.
3. Arrange the eggplant cubes on the baking sheet, then brush with 2 tablespoons of the balsamic vinegar mixture on both sides.
4. Broil in the preheated oven for 8 minutes or until lightly browned. Flip the cubes halfway through the cooking time.
5. Meanwhile, combine the chickpeas, mint, onion, garlic, and sesame seeds in a large serving bowl. Drizzle with remaining balsamic vinegar mixture. Stir to mix well.
6. Remove the eggplant from the oven. Allow to cool for 5 minutes, then slice them into ½-inch strips on a clean work surface.
7. Add the eggplant strips in the serving bowl, then toss to combine well before serving.

Cherry, Apricot, and Pecan Brown Rice Bowl

Prep time: 15 minutes | Cook time: 1 hour 1 minutes
Serves 2

2 tablespoons olive oil
2 green onions, sliced
½ cup brown rice
1 cup low -sodium chicken stock
2 tablespoons dried cherries
4 dried apricots, chopped
2 tablespoons pecans, toasted and chopped
Sea salt and freshly ground pepper, to taste

1. Heat the olive oil in a medium saucepan over medium-high heat until shimmering.
2. Add the green onions and sauté for 1 minutes or until fragrant.
3. Add the rice. Stir to mix well, then pour in the chicken stock.
4. Bring to a boil. Reduce the heat to low. Cover and simmer for 50 minutes or until the brown rice is soft.
5. Add the cherries, apricots, and pecans, and simmer for 10 more minutes or until the fruits are tender.
6. Pour them in a large serving bowl. Fluff with a fork. Sprinkle with sea salt and freshly ground pepper. Serve immediately.

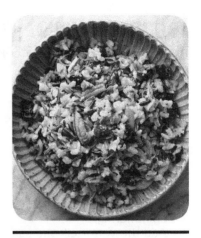

Tip: How to toast the pecans: Put the pecans in a skillet and heat over medium heat or until golden brown and toasted. Stir constantly.

Per Serving
calories: 451 | fat: 25.9g
protein: 8.2g | carbs: 50.4g
fiber: 4.6g | sodium: 122mg

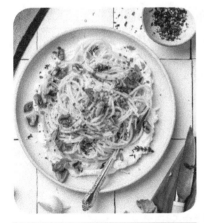

Tip: How to cook the spaghetti: Bring a large pot of water to a boil, then add the spaghetti and cook for 10 minutes or until al dente. Drain the spaghetti in a colander before using.

Per Serving
calories: 264 | fat: 16.8g
protein: 8.6g | carbs: 22.8g
fiber: 4.0g | sodium: 336mg

Easy Walnut and Ricotta Spaghetti

Prep time: 15 minutes | Cook time: 10 minutes
Serves 6

30m or less

1 pound (454 g) cooked whole-wheat spaghetti
2 tablespoons extra-virgin olive oil
4 cloves garlic, minced
¾ cup walnuts, toasted and finely chopped
2 tablespoons ricotta cheese
¼ cup flat-leaf parsley, chopped
½ cup grated Parmesan cheese
Sea salt and freshly ground pepper, to taste

1. Reserve a cup of spaghetti water while cooking the spaghetti.
2. Heat the olive oil in a nonstick skillet over medium-low heat or until shimmering.
3. Add the garlic and sauté for a minute or until fragrant.
4. Pour the spaghetti water into the skillet and cook for 8 more minutes.
5. Turn off the heat and mix in the walnuts and ricotta cheese.
6. Put the cooked spaghetti on a large serving plate, then pour the walnut sauce over. Spread with parsley and Parmesan, then sprinkle with salt and ground pepper. Toss to serve.

Lebanese Flavor Broken Thin Noodles

Prep time: 10 minutes | Cook time: 25 minutes
Serves 6

1 tablespoon extra-virgin olive oil
1 (3-ounce / 85-g) cup vermicelli, broken into 1- to 1½-inch pieces
3 cups shredded cabbage
1 cup brown rice
3 cups low-sodium vegetable soup

½ cup water
2 garlic cloves, mashed
¼ teaspoon sea salt
⅛ teaspoon crushed red pepper flakes
½ cup coarsely chopped cilantro
Fresh lemon slices, for serving

1. Heat the olive oil in a saucepan over medium-high heat until shimmering.
2. Add the vermicelli and sauté for 3 minutes or until toasted.
3. Add the cabbage and sauté for 4 minutes or until tender.
4. Pour in the brown rice, vegetable soup, and water. Add the garlic and sprinkle with salt and red pepper flakes.
5. Bring to a boil over high heat. Reduce the heat to medium low. Put the lid on and simmer for another 10 minutes.
6. Turn off the heat, then let sit for 5 minutes without opening the lid.
7. Pour them on a large serving platter and spread with cilantro. Squeeze the lemon slices over and serve warm.

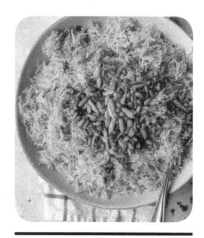

Tip: Instead of vermicelli, you can also use thin spaghetti.

Per Serving
calories: 127 | fat: 3.1g
protein: 4.2g | carbs: 22.9g
fiber: 3.0g | sodium: 224mg

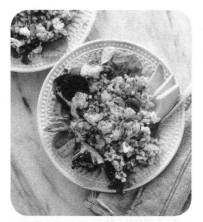

Tip: You can use a citrus zester to zest the lemon, then cut the lemon into wedges and squeeze the lemon juice over the farro bowl.

Per Serving
calories: 210 | fat: 11.1g
protein: 4.2g | carbs: 27.9g
fiber: 7.0g | sodium: 152mg

Lemony Farro and Avocado Bowl

Prep time: 5 minutes | Cook time: 25 minutes
Serves 4

30m or less

1 tablespoon plus 2 teaspoons extra-virgin olive oil, divided
½ medium onion, chopped
1 carrot, shredded
2 garlic cloves, minced
1 (6-ounce / 170-g) cup pearled farro
2 cups low-sodium vegetable soup
2 avocados, peeled, pitted, and sliced
Zest and juice of 1 small lemon
¼ teaspoon sea salt

1. Heat 1 tablespoon of olive oil in a saucepan over medium-high heat until shimmering.
2. Add the onion and sauté for 5 minutes or until translucent.
3. Add the carrot and garlic and sauté for 1 minute or until fragrant.
4. Add the farro and pour in the vegetable soup. Bring to a boil over high heat. Reduce the heat to low. Put the lid on and simmer for 20 minutes or until the farro is al dente.
5. Transfer the farro in a large serving bowl, then fold in the avocado slices. Sprinkle with lemon zest and salt, then drizzle with lemon juice and 2 teaspoons of olive oil.
6. Stir to mix well and serve immediately.

Rice and Blueberry Stuffed Sweet Potatoes

Prep time: 15 minutes | Cook time: 20 minutes
Serves 4

2 cups cooked wild rice
½ cup dried blueberries
½ cup chopped hazelnuts
½ cup shredded Swiss chard
1 teaspoon chopped fresh thyme
1 scallion, white and green parts, peeled and thinly sliced
Sea salt and freshly ground black pepper, to taste
4 sweet potatoes, baked in the skin until tender

1. Preheat the oven to 400ºF (205ºC).
2. Combine all the ingredients, except for the sweet potatoes, in a large bowl. Stir to mix well.
3. Cut the top third of the sweet potato off length wire, then scoop most of the sweet potato flesh out.
4. Fill the potato with the wild rice mixture, then set the sweet potato on a greased baking sheet.
5. Bake in the preheated oven for 20 minutes or until the sweet potato skin is lightly charred.
6. Serve immediately.

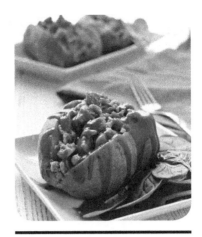

Tip: You can mix the sweet potato flesh in the bowl of wild rice mixture and fill them back in the sweet potato skin.

Per Serving
calories: 393 | fat: 7.1g
protein: 10.2g | carbs: 76.9g
fiber: 10.0g | sodium: 93mg

Slow Cooked Turkey and Brown Rice

Prep time: 20 minutes | Cook time: 3 hours 10 minutes
Serves 6

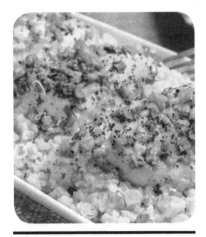

Tip: There are four types of brown rice, long grain, medium grain, short grain, and light brown rice. I prefer the long-grain brown rice, because it has a chewy texture and nutty flavor which is perfect for this dish.

Per Serving
calories: 499 | fat: 16.4g
protein: 32.4g | carbs: 56.5g
fiber: 4.7g | sodium: 758mg

1 tablespoon extra-virgin olive oil
1½ pounds (680 g) ground turkey
2 tablespoons chopped fresh sage, divided
2 tablespoons chopped fresh thyme, divided
1 teaspoon sea salt
½ teaspoon ground black pepper
2 cups brown rice
1 (14-ounce / 397-g) can stewed tomatoes, with the juice
¼ cup pitted and sliced Kalamata olives
3 medium zucchini, sliced thinly
¼ cup chopped fresh flat-leaf parsley
1 medium yellow onion, chopped
1 tablespoon plus 1 teaspoon balsamic vinegar
2 cups low-sodium chicken stock
2 garlic cloves, minced
½ cup grated Parmesan cheese, for serving

1. Heat the olive oil in a nonstick skillet over medium-high heat until shimmering.
2. Add the ground turkey and sprinkle with 1 tablespoon of sage, 1 tablespoon of thyme, salt and ground black pepper.
3. Sauté for 10 minutes or until the ground turkey is lightly browned.
4. Pour them in the slow cooker, then pour in the remaining ingredients, except for the Parmesan. Stir to mix well.
5. Put the lid on and cook on high for 3 hours or until the rice and vegetables are tender.
6. Pour them in a large serving bowl, then spread with Parmesan cheese before serving.

Papaya, Jicama, and Peas Rice Bowl

Prep time: 20 minutes | Cook time: 45 minutes
Serves 4

Sauce:

Juice of ¼ lemon
2 teaspoons chopped fresh basil
1 tablespoon raw honey

1 tablespoon extra-virgin olive oil
Sea salt, to taste

Rice:

1½ cups wild rice
2 papayas, peeled, seeded, and diced
1 jicama, peeled and shredded

1 cup snow peas, julienned
2 cups shredded cabbage
1 scallion, white and green parts, chopped

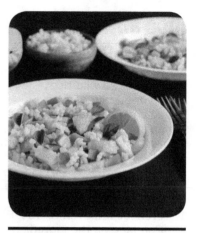

1. Combine the ingredients for the sauce in a bowl. Stir to mix well. Set aside until ready to use.
2. Pour the wild rice in a saucepan, then pour in enough water to cover. Bring to a boil.
3. Reduce the heat to low, then simmer for 45 minutes or until the wild rice is soft and plump. Drain and transfer to a large serving bowl.
4. Top the rice with papayas, jicama, peas, cabbage, and scallion. Pour the sauce over and stir to mix well before serving.

Tip: Instead of papaya, you can also use pineapple, peaches, apples, or cherry tomatoes.

Per Serving
calories: 446 | fat: 7.9g
protein: 13.1g | carbs: 85.8g
fiber: 16.0g | sodium: 70mg

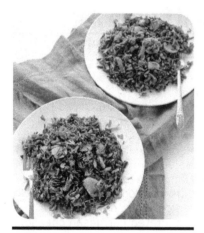

Tip: To make this a complete meal, you can serve it with seared tuna, or salmon casserole.

Per Serving
calories: 214 | fat: 3.9g
protein: 7.2g | carbs: 37.9g
fiber: 5.0g | sodium: 122mg

Wild Rice, Celery, and Cauliflower Pilaf

Prep time: 10 minutes | Cook time: 45 minutes
Serves 4

1 tablespoon olive oil, plus more for greasing the baking dish
1 cup wild rice
2 cups low-sodium chicken broth
1 sweet onion, chopped
2 stalks celery, chopped
1 teaspoon minced garlic

2 carrots, peeled, halved lengthwise, and sliced
½ cauliflower head, cut into small florets
1 teaspoon chopped fresh thyme
Sea salt, to taste

1. Preheat the oven to 350ºF (180ºC). Line a baking sheet with parchment paper and grease with olive oil.
2. Put the wild rice in a saucepan, then pour in the chicken broth. Bring to a boil. Reduce the heat to low and simmer for 30 minutes or until the rice is plump.
3. Meanwhile, heat the remaining olive oil in an oven-proof skillet over medium-high heat until shimmering.
4. Add the onion, celery, and garlic to the skillet and sauté for 3 minutes or until the onion is translucent.
5. Add the carrots and cauliflower to the skillet and sauté for 5 minutes. Turn off the heat and set aside.
6. Pour the cooked rice in the skillet with the vegetables. Sprinkle with thyme and salt.
7. Set the skillet in the preheated oven and bake for 15 minutes or until the vegetables are soft.
8. Serve immediately.

Curry Apple Couscous with Leeks and Pecans

Prep time: 10 minutes | Cook time: 8 minutes
Serves 4

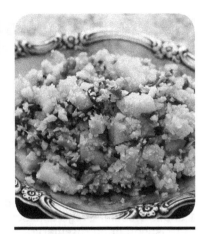

2 teaspoons extra-virgin olive oil
2 leeks, white parts only, sliced
1 apple, diced
2 cups cooked couscous
2 tablespoons curry powder
½ cup chopped pecans

1. Heat the olive oil in a skillet over medium heat until shimmering.
2. Add the leeks and sauté for 5 minutes or until soft.
3. Add the diced apple and cook for 3 more minutes until tender.
4. Add the couscous and curry powder. Stir to combine.
5. Transfer them in a large serving bowl, then mix in the pecans and serve.

Tip: How to cook the couscous: Bring a pot of water to a bowl, then sprinkle with salt and olive oil, if desired. Turn off the heat and pour the couscous in the pot. Cover and let sit for 10 minutes or until the couscous is tender.

Per Serving
calories: 254 | fat: 11.9g
protein: 5.4g | carbs: 34.3g
fiber: 5.9g | sodium: 15mg

Roasted Butternut Squash and Zucchini with Penne

Prep time: 15 minutes | Cook time: 30 minutes
Serves 6

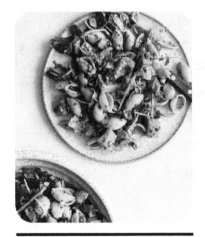

Tip: Instead of dry white wine, you can use the same amount of low-sodium chicken broth to replace it.

Per Serving
calories: 340 | fat: 6.2g
protein: 8.0g | carbs: 66.8g
fiber: 9.1g | sodium: 297mg

1 large zucchini, diced
1 large butternut squash, peeled and diced
1 large yellow onion, chopped
2 tablespoons extra-virgin olive oil
1 teaspoon paprika
½ teaspoon garlic powder
½ teaspoon sea salt
½ teaspoon freshly ground black pepper
1 pound (454 g) whole-grain penne
½ cup dry white wine
2 tablespoons grated Parmesan cheese

1. Preheat the oven to 400ºF (205ºC). Line a baking sheet with aluminum foil.
2. Combine the zucchini, butternut squash, and onion in a large bowl. Drizzle with olive oil and sprinkle with paprika, garlic powder, salt, and ground black pepper. Toss to coat well.
3. Spread the vegetables in the single layer on the baking sheet, then roast in the preheated oven for 25 minutes or until the vegetables are tender.
4. Meanwhile, bring a pot of water to a boil, then add the penne and cook for 14 minutes or until al dente. Drain the penne through a colander.
5. Transfer ½ cup of roasted vegetables in a food processor, then pour in the dry white wine. Pulse until smooth.
6. Pour the puréed vegetables in a nonstick skillet and cook with penne over medium-high heat for a few minutes to heat through.
7. Transfer the penne with the purée on a large serving plate, then spread the remaining roasted vegetables and Parmesan on top before serving.

Minestrone Chickpeas and Macaroni Casserole

Prep time: 20 minutes | Cook time: 7 hours 20 minutes
Serves 5

1 (15-ounce / 425-g) can chickpeas, drained and rinsed
1 (28-ounce / 794-g) can diced tomatoes, with the juice
1 (6-ounce / 170-g) can no-salt-added tomato paste
3 medium carrots, sliced
3 cloves garlic, minced
1 medium yellow onion, chopped
1 cup low-sodium vegetable soup
½ teaspoon dried rosemary

1 teaspoon dried oregano
2 teaspoons maple syrup
½ teaspoon sea salt
¼ teaspoon ground black pepper
½ pound (227-g) fresh green beans, trimmed and cut into bite-size pieces
1 cup macaroni pasta
2 ounces (57 g) Parmesan cheese, grated

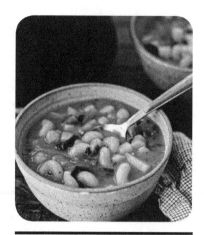

1. Except for the green beans, pasta, and Parmesan cheese, combine all the ingredients in the slow cooker and stir to mix well.
2. Put the slow cooker lid on and cook on low for 7 hours.
3. Fold in the pasta and green beans. Put the lid on and cook on high for 20 minutes or until the vegetable are soft and the pasta is al dente.
4. Pour them in a large serving bowl and spread with Parmesan cheese before serving.

Tip: Instead of chickpeas, you can also use kidney beans, great northern beans, or cannellini beans.

Per Serving
calories: 349 | fat: 6.7g
protein: 16.5g | carbs: 59.9g
fiber: 12.9g | sodium: 937mg

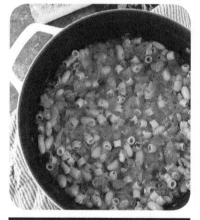

Tip: You can use the small whole-wheat pasta like penne, farfalle, shell, corkscrew, macaroni, or alphabet pasta.

Per Serving
calories: 357 | fat: 7.6g
protein: 18.2g | carbs: 64.5g
fiber: 10.1g | sodium: 454mg

Small Pasta and Beans Pot

Prep time: 20 minutes | Cook time: 15 minutes
Serves 2 to 4

1 pound (454 g) small whole wheat pasta
1 (14.5-ounce / 411-g) can diced tomatoes, juice reserved
1 (15-ounce / 425-g) can cannellini beans, drained and rinsed
2 tablespoons no-salt-added tomato paste
1 red or yellow bell pepper, chopped
1 yellow onion, chopped
1 tablespoon Italian seasoning mix
3 garlic cloves, minced
¼ teaspoon crushed red pepper flakes, optional
1 tablespoon extra-virgin olive oil
5 cups water
1 bunch kale, stemmed and chopped
½ cup pitted Kalamata olives, chopped
1 cup sliced basil

1. Except for the kale, olives, and basil, combine all the ingredients in a pot. Stir to mix well. Bring to a boil over high heat. Stir constantly.
2. Reduce the heat to medium high and add the kale. Cook for 10 minutes or until the pasta is al dente. Stir constantly.
3. Transfer all of them on a large plate and serve with olives and basil on top.

Swoodles with Almond Butter Sauce

Prep time: 20 minutes | Cook time: 20 minutes
Serves 4

Sauce:
1 garlic clove
1-inch piece fresh ginger, peeled and sliced
¼ cup chopped yellow onion
¾ cup almond butter
1 tablespoon tamari
1 tablespoon raw honey
1 teaspoon paprika
1 tablespoon fresh lemon juice
⅛ teaspoon ground red pepper
Sea salt and ground black pepper, to taste
¼ cup water

Swoodles:
2 large sweet potatoes, spiralized
2 tablespoons coconut oil, melted
Sea salt and ground black pepper, to taste

For Serving:
½ cup fresh parsley, chopped
½ cup thinly sliced scallions

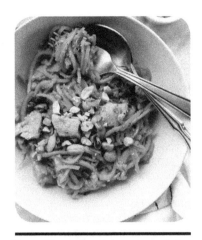

Tips: To make this a complete meal, you can serve it along with cashew slaw.
You can use the store-bought swoodles or spiralize the sweet potatoes with spiralizer yourself.

Per Serving
calories: 441 | fat: 33.6g
protein: 12.0g | carbs: 29.6g
fiber: 7.8g | sodium: 479mg

Make the Sauce
1. Put the garlic, ginger, and onion in a food processor, then pulse to combine well.
2. Add the almond butter, tamari, honey, paprika, lemon juice, ground red pepper, salt, and black pepper to the food processor. Pulse to combine well. Pour in the water during the pulsing until the mixture is thick and smooth.

Make the Swoodles:
1. Preheat the oven to 425ºF (220ºC). Line a baking sheet with parchment paper.
2. Put the spiralized sweet potato in a bowl, then drizzle with olive oil. Toss to coat well. Transfer them on the baking sheet. Sprinkle with salt and pepper.
3. Bake in the preheated oven for 20 minutes or until lightly browned and al dente. Check the doneness during the baking and remove any well-cooked swoodles.
4. Transfer the swoodles on a large plate and spread with sauce, parsley, and scallions. Toss to serve.

Spicy Italian Bean Balls with Marinara

Prep time: 20 minutes | Cook time: 30 minutes
Serves 2 to 4

Bean Balls:
1 tablespoon extra-virgin olive oil
½ yellow onion, minced
1 teaspoon fennel seeds
2 teaspoons dried oregano
½ teaspoon crushed red pepper flakes
1 teaspoon garlic powder
1 (15-ounce / 425-g) can white beans (cannellini or navy), drained and rinsed
½ cup whole-grain bread crumbs
Sea salt and ground black pepper, to taste

Marinara:
1 tablespoon extra-virgin olive oil
3 garlic cloves, minced
Handful basil leaves
1 (28-ounce / 794-g) can chopped tomatoes with juice reserved
Sea salt, to taste

Make the Bean Balls
1. Preheat the oven to 350°F (180°C). Line a baking sheet with parchment paper.
2. Heat the olive oil in a nonstick skillet over medium heat until shimmering.
3. Add the onion and sauté for 5 minutes or until translucent.
4. Sprinkle with fennel seeds, oregano, red pepper flakes, and garlic powder, then cook for 1 minute or until aromatic.
5. Pour the sautéed mixture in a food processor and add the beans and bread crumbs. Sprinkle with salt and ground black pepper, then pulse to combine well and the mixture holds together.
6. Shape the mixture into balls with a 2-ounce (57-g) cookie scoop, then arrange the balls on the baking sheet.
7. Bake in the preheated oven for 30 minutes or until lightly browned. Flip the balls halfway through the cooking time.

Make the Marinara
1. While baking the bean balls, heat the olive oil in a saucepan over medium-high heat until shimmering.
2. Add the garlic and basil and sauté for 2 minutes or until fragrant.
3. Fold in the tomatoes and juice. Bring to a boil. Reduce the heat to low. Put the lid on and simmer for 15 minutes. Sprinkle with salt.
4. Transfer the bean balls on a large plate and baste with marinara before serving.

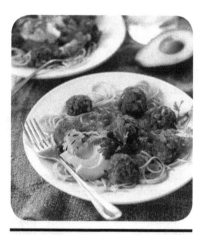

Tips: Wet your hands while shaping the bean balls to avoid sticking.
To make this a complete meal, you can serve the balls and the sauce with all kinds of cooked pasta, such as pappardelle pasta, corkscrew pasta, farfalle pasta, or shell pasta.

Per Serving
calories: 351 | fat: 16.4g
protein: 11.5g | carbs: 42.9g
fiber: 10.3g | sodium: 377mg

Hearty Butternut Spinach, and Cheeses Lasagna

Prep time: 30 minutes | Cook time: 3 hours 45 minutes
Serves 4 to 6

2 tablespoons extra-virgin olive oil, divided
1 butternut squash, halved lengthwise and deseeded
½ teaspoon sage
½ teaspoon sea salt
¼ teaspoon ground black pepper
¼ cup grated Parmesan cheese
2 cups ricotta cheese
½ cup unsweetened almond milk
5 layers whole-wheat lasagna noodles (about 12 ounces / 340 g in total)
4 ounces (113 g) fresh spinach leaves, divided
½ cup shredded part skim Mozzarella, for garnish

1. Preheat the oven to 400ºF (205ºC). Line a baking sheet with parchment paper.
2. Brush 1 tablespoon of olive oil on the cut side of the butternut squash, then place the squash on the baking sheet.
3. Bake in the preheated oven for 45 minutes or until the squash is tender.
4. Allow to cool until you can handle it, then scoop the flesh out and put the flesh in a food processor to purée.
5. Combine the puréed butternut squash flesh with sage, salt, and ground black pepper in a large bowl. Stir to mix well.
6. Combine the cheeses and milk in a separate bowl, then sprinkle with salt and pepper, to taste.
7. Grease the slow cooker with 1 tablespoon of olive oil, then add a layer of lasagna noodles to coat the bottom of the slow cooker.
8. Spread half of the squash mixture on top of the noodles, then top the squash mixture with another layer of lasagna noodles.
9. Spread half of the spinach over the noodles, then top the spinach with half of cheese mixture. Repeat with remaining 3 layers of lasagna noodles, squash mixture, spinach, and cheese mixture.
10. Top the cheese mixture with Mozzarella, then put the lid on and cook on low for 3 hours or until the lasagna noodles are al dente.
11. Serve immediately.

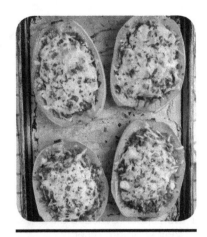

Tip: To make this a complete meal, you can serve it with fresh cucumber soup and green leafy salad.

Per Serving
calories: 657 | fat: 37.1g
protein: 30.9g | carbs: 57.2g
fiber: 8.3g | sodium: 918mg

Rich Cauliflower Alfredo

Prep time: 35 minutes | Cook time: 30 minutes
Serves 4

Cauliflower Alfredo Sauce:
1 tablespoon avocado oil
½ yellow onion, diced
2 cups cauliflower florets
2 garlic cloves, minced
1½ teaspoons miso
1 teaspoon Dijon mustard

Pinch of ground nutmeg
½ cup unsweetened almond milk
1½ tablespoons fresh lemon juice
2 tablespoons nutritional yeast
Sea salt and ground black pepper, to taste

Fettuccine:
1 tablespoon avocado oil
½ yellow onion, diced
1 cup broccoli florets
1 zucchini, halved lengthwise and cut into ¼-inch-thick half-moons
Sea salt and ground black pepper, to taste
½ cup sun-dried tomatoes, drained if packed in oil
8 ounces (227 g) cooked whole-wheat fettuccine
½ cup fresh basil, cut into ribbons

Make the Sauce:
1. Heat the avocado oil in a nonstick skillet over medium-high heat until shimmering.
2. Add half of the onion to the skillet and sauté for 5 minutes or until translucent.
3. Add the cauliflower and garlic to the skillet. Reduce the heat to low and cook for 8 minutes or until the cauliflower is tender.
4. Pour them in a food processor, add the remaining ingredients for the sauce and pulse to combine well. Set aside.

Make the Fettuccine:
1. Heat the avocado oil in a nonstick skillet over medium-high heat.
2. Add the remaining half of onion and sauté for 5 minutes or until translucent.
3. Add the broccoli and zucchini. Sprinkle with salt and ground black pepper, then sauté for 5 minutes or until tender.
4. Add the sun-dried tomatoes, reserved sauce, and fettuccine. Sauté for 3 minutes or until well-coated and heated through.
5. Serve the fettuccine on a large plate and spread with basil before serving.

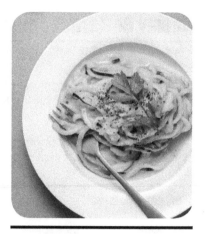

Tip: How to cook the fettuccine: Bring a large pot of water to a boil, then add the fettuccine and cook for 8 minutes or until al dente. Drain the fettuccine in a colander before using.

Per Serving
calories: 288 | fat: 15.9g
protein: 10.1g | carbs: 32.5g
fiber: 8.1g | sodium: 185mg

Fried Eggplant Rolls

Prep time: 20 minutes | Cook time: 10 minutes
Serves 4 to 6

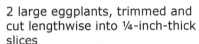

2 large eggplants, trimmed and cut lengthwise into ¼-inch-thick slices
1 teaspoon salt
1 cup shredded ricotta cheese
4 ounces (113 g) goat cheese, shredded
¼ cup finely chopped fresh basil
½ teaspoon freshly ground black pepper
Olive oil spray

1. Add the eggplant slices to a colander and season with salt. Set aside for 15 to 20 minutes.
2. Mix together the ricotta and goat cheese, basil, and black pepper in a large bowl and stir to combine. Set aside.
3. Dry the eggplant slices with paper towels and lightly mist them with olive oil spray.
4. Heat a large skillet over medium heat and lightly spray it with olive oil spray.
5. Arrange the eggplant slices in the skillet and fry each side for 3 minutes until golden brown.
6. Remove from the heat to a paper towel-lined plate and rest for 5 minutes.
7. Make the eggplant rolls: Lay the eggplant slices on a flat work surface and top each slice with a tablespoon of the prepared cheese mixture. Roll them up and serve immediately.

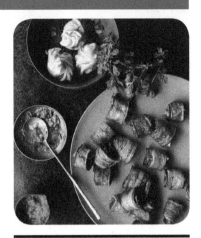

Tips: The eggplant rolls can be made in advance and stored in the refrigerator. You can add 1 teaspoon of lemon zest to the filling for a punch of citrus flavor.

Per Serving
calories: 254 | fat: 14.9g
protein: 15.3g | carbs: 18.6g
fiber: 7.1g | sodium: 745mg

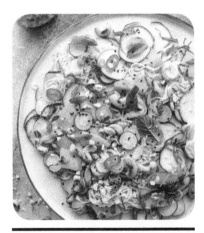

Tip: For different flavors, you can grill, fry, or even roast the zucchini. The mint can be replaced with the oregano in this recipe.

Per Serving
calories: 146 | fat: 10.6g
protein: 4.2g | carbs: 11.8g
fiber: 3.0g | sodium: 606mg

Garlicky Zucchini Cubes with Mint

Prep time: 5 minutes | Cook time: 10 minutes
Serves 4

3 large green zucchini, cut into ½-inch cubes
3 tablespoons extra-virgin olive oil
1 large onion, chopped
3 cloves garlic, minced
1 teaspoon salt
1 teaspoon dried mint

1. Heat the olive oil in a large skillet over medium heat.
2. Add the onion and garlic and sauté for 3 minutes, stirring constantly, or until softened.
3. Stir in the zucchini cubes and salt and cook for 5 minutes, or until the zucchini is browned and tender.
4. Add the mint to the skillet and toss to combine, then continue cooking for 2 minutes.
5. Serve warm.

Cauliflower Hash with Carrots

Prep time: 10 minutes | Cook time: 10 minutes
Serves 4

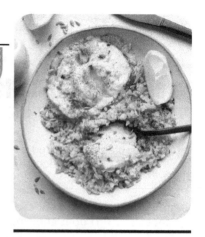

3 tablespoons extra-virgin olive oil
1 large onion, chopped
1 tablespoon minced garlic

2 cups diced carrots
4 cups cauliflower florets
½ teaspoon ground cumin
1 teaspoon salt

1. In a large skillet, heat the olive oil over medium heat.
2. Add the onion and garlic and sauté for 1 minute. Stir in the carrots and stir-fry for 3 minutes.
3. Add the cauliflower florets, cumin, and salt and toss to combine.
4. Cover and cook for 3 minutes until lightly browned. Stir well and cook, uncovered, for 3 to 4 minutes, until softened.
5. Remove from the heat and serve warm.

Tip: For an even heartier dish, serve the vegetable hash with whole-grain pasta or rice.

Per Serving
calories: 158 | fat: 10.8g
protein: 3.1g | carbs: 14.9g
fiber: 5.1g | sodium: 656mg

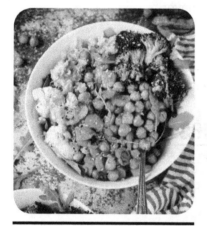

Tip: If you like the Brussels sprouts, you can add them to this dish. Slice the Brussels sprouts in half and roast them with the vegetables in the preheated oven.

Per Serving
calories: 453 | fat: 17.8g
protein: 12.1g | carbs: 61.8g
fiber: 11.2g | sodium: 60mg

Roasted Veggies and Brown Rice Bowl

Prep time: 15 minutes | Cook time: 20 minutes
Serves 4

2 cups cauliflower florets
2 cups broccoli florets
1 (15-ounce / 425-g) can chickpeas, drained and rinsed
1 cup carrot slices (about 1 inch thick)
2 to 3 tablespoons extra-virgin

olive oil, divided
Salt and freshly ground black pepper, to taste
Nonstick cooking spray
2 cups cooked brown rice
2 to 3 tablespoons sesame seeds, for garnish

Dressing:
3 to 4 tablespoons tahini
2 tablespoons honey
1 lemon, juiced

1 garlic clove, minced
Salt and freshly ground black pepper, to taste

1. Preheat the oven to 400ºF (205ºC). Spritz two baking sheets with nonstick cooking spray.
2. Spread the cauliflower and broccoli on the first baking sheet and the second with the chickpeas and carrot slices.
3. Drizzle each sheet with half of the olive oil and sprinkle with salt and pepper. Toss to coat well.
4. Roast the chickpeas and carrot slices in the preheated oven for 10 minutes, leaving the carrots tender but crisp, and the cauliflower and broccoli for 20 minutes until fork-tender. Stir them once halfway through the cooking time.
5. Meanwhile, make the dressing: Whisk together the tahini, honey, lemon juice, garlic, salt, and pepper in a small bowl.
6. Divide the cooked brown rice among four bowls. Top each bowl evenly with roasted vegetables and dressing. Sprinkle the sesame seeds on top for garnish before serving.

Zucchini and Artichokes Bowl with Farro

Prep time: 15 minutes | Cook time: 10 minutes
Serves 4 to 6

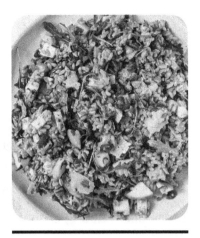

1/3 cup extra-virgin olive oil
1/3 cup chopped red onions
½ cup chopped red bell pepper
2 garlic cloves, minced
1 cup zucchini, cut into ½-inch-thick slices
½ cup coarsely chopped artichokes
½ cup canned chickpeas, drained and rinsed
3 cups cooked farro

Salt and freshly ground black pepper, to taste
½ cup crumbled feta cheese, for serving (optional)
¼ cup sliced olives, for serving (optional)
2 tablespoons fresh basil, chiffonade, for serving (optional)
3 tablespoons balsamic vinegar, for serving (optional)

1. Heat the olive oil in a large skillet over medium heat until it shimmers.
2. Add the onions, bell pepper, and garlic and sauté for 5 minutes, stirring occasionally, until softened.
3. Stir in the zucchini slices, artichokes, and chickpeas and sauté for about 5 minutes until slightly tender.
4. Add the cooked farro and toss to combine until heated through. Sprinkle the salt and pepper to season.
5. Divide the mixture into bowls. Top each bowl evenly with feta cheese, olive slices, and basil and sprinkle with the balsamic vinegar, if desired.

Tip: You can replace the farro with your favorite gluten-free base.

Per Serving
calories: 366 | fat: 19.9g
protein: 9.3g | carbs: 50.7g
fiber: 9.0g | sodium: 86mg

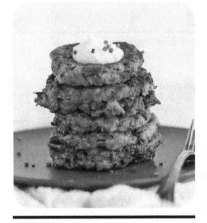

Tip: You can add any of your favorite herbs such as basil, thyme, or parsley to the zucchini mixture.

Per Serving (2 fritters)
calories: 113 | fat: 6.1g
protein: 4.0g | carbs: 12.2g
fiber: 1.0g | sodium: 25mg

5-Ingredient Zucchini Fritters

Prep time: 15 minutes | Cook time: 5 minutes
Makes 14 fritters

4 cups grated zucchini
Salt, to taste
2 large eggs, lightly beaten
1/3 cup sliced scallions (green and white parts)
2/3 all-purpose flour
⅛ teaspoon black pepper
2 tablespoons olive oil

1. Put the grated zucchini in a colander and lightly season with salt. Set aside to rest for 10 minutes. Squeeze out as much liquid from the grated zucchini as possible.
2. Pour the grated zucchini into a bowl. Fold in the beaten eggs, scallions, flour, salt, and pepper and stir until everything is well combined.
3. Heat the olive oil in a large skillet over medium heat until hot.
4. Drop 3 tablespoons mounds of the zucchini mixture onto the hot skillet to make each fritter, pressing them lightly into rounds and spacing them about 2 inches apart.
5. Cook for 2 to 3 minutes. Flip the zucchini fritters and cook for 2 minutes more, or until they are golden brown and cooked through.
6. Remove from the heat to a plate lined with paper towels. Repeat with the remaining zucchini mixture.
7. Serve hot.

Moroccan Tagine with Vegetables

Prep time: 20 minutes | Cook time: 40 minutes
Serves 2

2 tablespoons olive oil
½ onion, diced
1 garlic clove, minced
2 cups cauliflower florets
1 medium carrot, cut into 1-inch pieces
1 cup diced eggplant
1 (28-ounce / 794-g) can whole tomatoes with their juices
1 (15-ounce / 425-g) can

chickpeas, drained and rinsed
2 small red potatoes, cut into 1-inch pieces
1 cup water
1 teaspoon pure maple syrup
½ teaspoon cinnamon
½ teaspoon turmeric
1 teaspoon cumin
½ teaspoon salt
1 to 2 teaspoons harissa paste

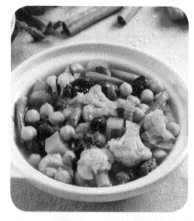

1. In a Dutch oven, heat the olive oil over medium-high heat. Sauté the onion for 5 minutes, stirring occasionally, or until the onion is translucent.
2. Stir in the garlic, cauliflower florets, carrot, eggplant, tomatoes, and potatoes. Using a wooden spoon or spatula to break up the tomatoes into smaller pieces.
3. Add the chickpeas, water, maple syrup, cinnamon, turmeric, cumin, and salt and stir to incorporate. Bring the mixture to a boil.
4. Once it starts to boil, reduce the heat to medium-low. Stir in the harissa paste, cover, allow to simmer for about 40 minutes, or until the vegetables are softened. Taste and adjust seasoning as needed.
5. Let the mixture cool for 5 minutes before serving.

Tip: A tagine is a corn-shaped cooking vessel traditionally used in Morocco. This recipe uses the Dutch oven that works just as well for this stew.

Per Serving
calories: 293 | fat: 9.9g
protein: 11.2g | carbs: 45.5g
fiber: 12.1g | sodium: 337mg

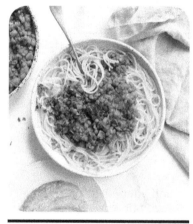

Tip: You can use 1 cup of cooked bulgur wheat or minced mushrooms to substitute for the lentils.

Per Serving
calories: 367 | fat: 15.0g
protein: 13.7g | carbs: 44.5g
fiber: 17.6g | sodium: 1108mg

Vegan Lentil Bolognese

Prep time: 15 minutes | Cook time: 50 minutes
Serves 2

1 medium celery stalk
1 large carrot
½ large onion
1 garlic clove
2 tablespoons olive oil
1 (28-ounce / 794-g) can crushed tomatoes
1 cup red wine
½ teaspoon salt, plus more as needed
½ teaspoon pure maple syrup
1 cup cooked lentils (prepared from ½ cup dry)

1. Add the celery, carrot, onion, and garlic to a food processor and process until everything is finely chopped.
2. In a Dutch oven, heat the olive oil over medium-high heat. Add the chopped mixture and sauté for about 10 minutes, stirring occasionally, or until the vegetables are lightly browned.
3. Stir in the tomatoes, wine, salt, and maple syrup and bring to a boil.
4. Once the sauce starts to boil, cover, and reduce the heat to medium-low. Simmer for 30 minutes, stirring occasionally, or until the vegetables are softened.
5. Stir in the cooked lentils and cook for an additional 5 minutes until warmed through.
6. Taste and add additional salt, if needed. Serve warm.

Grilled Vegetable Skewers

Prep time: 15 minutes | Cook time: 10 minutes
Serves 4

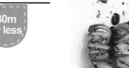

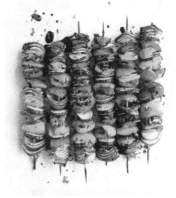

4 medium red onions, peeled and sliced into 6 wedges
4 medium zucchini, cut into 1-inch-thick slices
2 beefsteak tomatoes, cut into quarters
4 red bell peppers, cut into 2-inch squares
2 orange bell peppers, cut into 2-inch squares
2 yellow bell peppers, cut into 2-inch squares
2 tablespoons plus 1 teaspoon olive oil, divided

SPECIAL EQUIPMENT:
4 wooden skewers, soaked in water for at least 30 minutes

1. Preheat the grill to medium-high heat.
2. Skewer the vegetables by alternating between red onion, zucchini, tomatoes, and the different colored bell peppers. Brush them with 2 tablespoons of olive oil.
3. Oil the grill grates with 1 teaspoon of olive oil and grill the vegetable skewers for 5 minutes. Flip the skewers and grill for 5 minutes more, or until they are cooked to your liking.
4. Let the skewers cool for 5 minutes before serving.

Tip: You can add any leftover vegetables to a pita with a dollop of hummus for a quick and easy lunch or dinner.

Per Serving
calories: 115 | fat: 3.0g
protein: 3.5g | carbs: 18.7g
fiber: 4.7g | sodium: 12mg

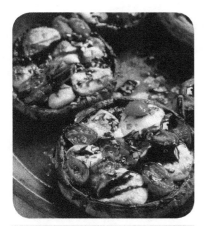

Tips: You can make a caprese mushroom cap by substituting your favorite jarred pesto sauce for the tomato sauce. And if you are a meat lover, add ½ pound (227 g) cooked, ground chicken to the filling.

Per Serving
calories: 217 | fat: 15.8g
protein: 11.2g | carbs: 11.7g
fiber: 2.0g | sodium: 243mg

Stuffed Portobello Mushroom with Tomatoes

Prep time: 10 minutes | Cook time: 15 minutes
Serves 4

4 large portobello mushroom caps
3 tablespoons extra-virgin olive oil
Salt and freshly ground black pepper, to taste
4 sun-dried tomatoes
1 cup shredded mozzarella cheese, divided
½ to ¾ cup low-sodium tomato sauce

1. Preheat the broiler on high.
2. Arrange the mushroom caps on a baking sheet and drizzle with olive oil. Sprinkle with salt and pepper.
3. Broil for 1o minutes, flipping the mushroom caps halfway through, until browned on the top.
4. Remove from the broil. Spoon 1 tomato, 2 tablespoons of cheese, and 2 to 3 tablespoons of sauce onto each mushroom cap.
5. Return the mushroom caps to the broiler and continue broiling for 2 to 3 minutes.
6. Cool for 5 minutes before serving.

Wilted Dandelion Greens with Sweet Onion

Prep time: 15 minutes | Cook time: 15 minutes
Serves 4

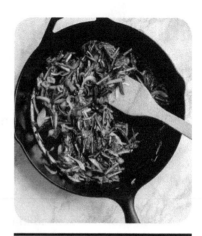

1 tablespoon extra-virgin olive oil
2 garlic cloves, minced
1 Vidalia onion, thinly sliced
½ cup low-sodium vegetable broth
2 bunches dandelion greens, roughly chopped
Freshly ground black pepper, to taste

1. Heat the olive oil in a large skillet over low heat.
2. Add the garlic and onion and cook for 2 to 3 minutes, stirring occasionally, or until the onion is translucent.
3. Fold in the vegetable broth and dandelion greens and cook for 5 to 7 minutes until wilted, stirring frequently.
4. Sprinkle with the black pepper and serve on a plate while warm.

Tip: For extra flavor and nutrition, you can add the dandelion greens to a white bean salad, soup or even stew. And the chili pepper also pairs perfectly with these greens.

Per Serving
calories: 81 | fat: 3.9g
protein: 3.2g | carbs: 10.8g
fiber: 4.0g | sodium: 72mg

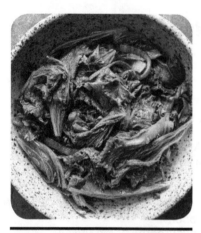

Celery and Mustard Greens

Prep time: 10 minutes | Cook time: 15 minutes
Serves 4

½ cup low-sodium vegetable broth
1 celery stalk, roughly chopped
½ sweet onion, chopped
½ large red bell pepper, thinly sliced
2 garlic cloves, minced
1 bunch mustard greens, roughly chopped

1. Pour the vegetable broth into a large cast iron pan and bring it to a simmer over medium heat.
2. Stir in the celery, onion, bell pepper, and garlic. Cook uncovered for about 3 to 5 minutes, or until the onion is softened.
3. Add the mustard greens to the pan and stir well. Cover, reduce the heat to low, and cook for an additional 10 minutes, or until the liquid is evaporated and the greens are wilted.
4. Remove from the heat and serve warm.

Tips: If the mustard greens aren't available, you can use the turnip greens. For added color and flavor, serve it with a sprinkle of red pepper flakes and a squeeze of lemon before serving.

Per Serving (1 cup)
calories: 39 | fat: 0g protein: 3.1g | carbs: 6.8g fiber: 3.0g | sodium: 120mg

Vegetable and Tofu Scramble

Prep time: 5 minutes | Cook time: 10 minutes
Serves 2

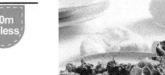
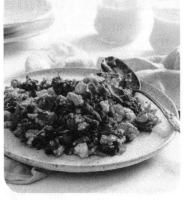

2 tablespoons extra-virgin olive oil
½ red onion, finely chopped
1 cup chopped kale
8 ounces (227 g) mushrooms, sliced
8 ounces (227 g) tofu, cut into pieces
2 garlic cloves, minced
Pinch red pepper flakes
½ teaspoon sea salt
⅛ teaspoon freshly ground black pepper

1. Heat the olive oil in a medium nonstick skillet over medium-high heat until shimmering.
2. Add the onion, kale, and mushrooms to the skillet and cook for about 5 minutes, stirring occasionally, or until the vegetables start to brown.
3. Add the tofu and stir-fry for 3 to 4 minutes until softened.
4. Stir in the garlic, red pepper flakes, salt, and black pepper and cook for 30 seconds.
5. Let the mixture cool for 5 minutes before serving.

Tip: If you'd like to add some carbs to this dish, you can serve the vegetable and tofu scramble over the whole-grain toast and pita bread.

Per Serving
calories: 233 | fat: 15.9g
protein: 13.4g | carbs: 11.9g
fiber: 2.0g | sodium: 672mg

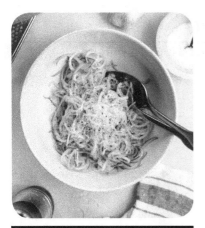

Simple Zoodles

Prep time: 10 minutes | Cook time: 5 minutes
Serves 2

2 tablespoons avocado oil
2 medium zucchini, spiralized
¼ teaspoon salt
Freshly ground black pepper, to taste

1. Heat the avocado oil in a large skillet over medium heat until it shimmers.
2. Add the zucchini noodles, salt, and black pepper to the skillet and toss to coat. Cook for 1 to 2 minutes, stirring constantly, until tender.
3. Serve warm.

Tips: Don't cook the zucchini noodles too long, or they will be not al dente. You can use a spiralizer, vegetable peeler, or sharp knife to make the zoodles.

Per Serving
calories: 128 | fat: 14.0g
protein: 0.3g | carbs: 0.3g
fiber: 0.1g | sodium: 291mg

Lentil and Tomato Collard Wraps

Prep time: 15 minutes | Cook time: 0 minutes
Serves 4

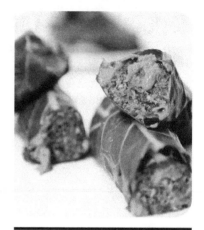

2 cups cooked lentils
5 Roma tomatoes, diced
½ cup crumbled feta cheese
10 large fresh basil leaves, thinly sliced
¼ cup extra-virgin olive oil
1 tablespoon balsamic vinegar
2 garlic cloves, minced
½ teaspoon raw honey
½ teaspoon salt
¼ teaspoon freshly ground black pepper
4 large collard leaves, stems removed

1. Combine the lentils, tomatoes, cheese, basil leaves, olive oil, vinegar, garlic, honey, salt, and black pepper in a large bowl and stir until well blended.
2. Lay the collard leaves on a flat work surface. Spoon the equal-sized amounts of the lentil mixture onto the edges of the leaves. Roll them up and slice in half to serve.

Tip: If you want to make the collard leaves easier to wrap, you can steam them for 1 to 2 minutes before wrapping.

Per Serving
calories: 318 | fat: 17.6g
protein: 13.2g | carbs: 27.5g
fiber: 9.9g | sodium: 475mg

Stir-Fry Baby Bok Choy

Prep time: 12 minutes | Cook time: 10 to 13 minutes
Serves 6

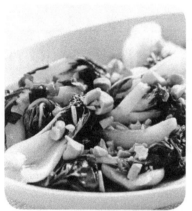

2 tablespoons coconut oil
1 large onion, finely diced
2 teaspoons ground cumin
1-inch piece fresh ginger, grated
1 teaspoon ground turmeric
½ teaspoon salt
12 baby bok choy heads, ends trimmed and sliced lengthwise
Water, as needed
3 cups cooked brown rice

1. Heat the coconut oil in a large pan over medium heat.
2. Sauté the onion for 5 minutes, stirring occasionally, or until the onion is translucent.
3. Fold in the cumin, ginger, turmeric, and salt and stir to coat well.
4. Add the bok choy and cook for 5 to 8 minutes, stirring occasionally, or until the bok choy is tender but crisp. You can add 1 tablespoon of water at a time, if the skillet gets dry until you finish sautéing.
5. Transfer the bok choy to a plate and serve over the cooked brown rice.

Tip: To add more flavors to this meal, you can serve this stir-fired bok choy with a simple grilled steak or harissa chicken.

Per Serving
calories: 443 | fat: 8.8g
protein: 30.3g | carbs: 75.7g
fiber: 19.0g | sodium: 1289mg

Sweet Pepper Stew

Prep time: 20 minutes | Cook time: 50 minutes
Serves 2

2 tablespoons olive oil
2 sweet peppers, diced (about 2 cups)
½ large onion, minced
1 garlic clove, minced
1 tablespoon gluten-free Worcestershire sauce

1 teaspoon oregano
1 cup low-sodium tomato juice
1 cup low-sodium vegetable stock
¼ cup brown rice
¼ cup brown lentils
Salt, to taste

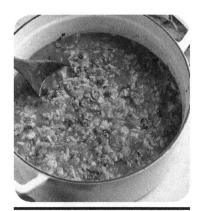

1. In a Dutch oven, heat the olive oil over medium-high heat.
2. Sauté the sweet peppers and onion for 10 minutes, stirring occasionally, or until the onion begins to turn golden and the peppers are wilted.
3. Stir in the garlic, Worcestershire sauce, and oregano and cook for 30 seconds more. Add the tomato juice, vegetable stock, rice, and lentils to the Dutch oven and stir to mix well.
4. Bring the mixture to a boil and then reduce the heat to medium-low. Let it simmer covered for about 45 minutes, or until the rice is cooked through and the lentils are tender.
5. Sprinkle with salt and serve warm.

Tips: If you'd like to use the meat in place of lentils, try adding lean ground turkey, beef, or lamb, and substitute the beef stock for vegetable stock. If the stew gets too thick, you can thin it with extra water to reach your preferred preference.

Per Serving
calories: 378 | fat: 15.6g
protein: 11.4g | carbs: 52.8g
fiber: 7.0g | sodium: 391mg

Vegetable and Red Lentil Stew

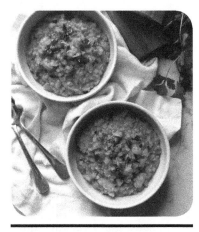

Prep time: 10 minutes | Cook time: 35 minutes
Serves 6

5-ingre

1 tablespoon extra-virgin olive oil
2 onions, peeled and finely diced
6½ cups water
2 zucchini, finely diced
4 celery stalks, finely diced
3 cups red lentils
1 teaspoon dried oregano
1 teaspoon salt, plus more as needed

1. Heat the olive oil in a large pot over medium heat.
2. Add the onions and sauté for about 5 minutes, stirring constantly, or until the onions are softened.
3. Stir in the water, zucchini, celery, lentils, oregano, and salt and bring the mixture to a boil.
4. Reduce the heat to low and let simmer covered for 30 minutes, stirring occasionally, or until the lentils are tender.
5. Taste and adjust the seasoning as needed.

Tip: You can try this recipe with different lentils such as brown and green lentils, but they need additional cooking time, about 20 minutes.

Per Serving
calories: 387 | fat: 4.4g
protein: 24.0g | carbs: 63.7g
fiber: 11.7g | sodium: 418mg

Roasted Vegetables

Prep time: 20 minutes | Cook time: 35 minutes
Serves 2

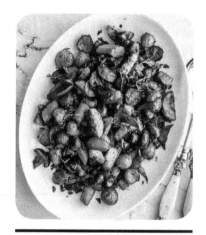

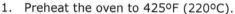

6 teaspoons extra-virgin olive oil, divided
12 to 15 Brussels sprouts, halved
1 medium sweet potato, peeled and cut into 2-inch cubes
2 cups fresh cauliflower florets
1 medium zucchini, cut into 1-inch rounds
1 red bell pepper, cut into 1-inch slices
Salt, to taste

1. Preheat the oven to 425ºF (220ºC).
2. Add 2 teaspoons of olive oil, Brussels sprouts, sweet potato, and salt to a large bowl and toss until they are completely coated.
3. Transfer them to a large roasting pan and roast for 10 minutes, or until the Brussels sprouts are lightly browned.
4. Meantime, combine the cauliflower florets with 2 teaspoons of olive oil and salt in a separate bowl.
5. Remove from the oven. Add the cauliflower florets to the roasting pan and roast for 10 minutes more.
6. Meanwhile, toss the zucchini and bell pepper with the remaining olive oil in a medium bowl until well coated. Season with salt.
7. Remove the roasting pan from the oven and stir in the zucchini and bell pepper. Continue roasting for 15 minutes, or until the vegetables are fork-tender.
8. Divide the roasted vegetables between two plates and serve warm.

Tip: To make this a complete meal, serve these roasted vegetables with grilled chicken, steak, or fish.

Per Serving
calories: 333 | fat: 16.8g
protein: 12.2g | carbs: 37.6g
fiber: 11.0g | sodium: 329mg

Ratatouille

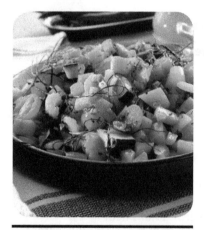

Prep time: 10 minutes | Cook time: 30 minutes
Serves 4

4 tablespoons extra-virgin olive oil, divided
1 cup diced zucchini
2 cups diced eggplant
1 cup diced onion
1 cup chopped green bell pepper
1 (15-ounce / 425-g) can no-salt-added diced tomatoes
½ teaspoon garlic powder
1 teaspoon ground thyme
Salt and freshly ground black pepper, to taste

1. Heat 2 tablespoons of olive oil in a large saucepan over medium heat until it shimmers.
2. Add the zucchini and eggplant and sauté for 10 minutes, stirring occasionally. If necessary, add the remaining olive oil.
3. Stir in the onion and bell pepper and sauté for 5 minutes until softened.
4. Add the diced tomatoes with their juice, garlic powder, and thyme and stir to combine. Continue cooking for 15 minutes until the vegetables are cooked through, stirring occasionally. Sprinkle with salt and black pepper.
5. Remove from the heat and serve on a plate.

Tips: For added protein, serve topped with shredded Parmesan cheese. To save time, you can use the frozen chopped green bell peppers.

Per Serving
calories: 189 | fat: 13.7g
protein: 3.1g | carbs: 14.8g
fiber: 4.0g | sodium: 27mg

Sautéed Green Beans with Tomatoes

Prep time: 10 minutes | Cook time: 20 minutes
Serves 4

 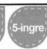

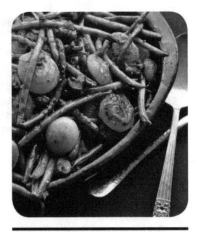

¼ cup extra-virgin olive oil
1 large onion, chopped
4 cloves garlic, finely chopped
1 pound (454 g) green beans, fresh or frozen, cut into 2-inch pieces
1½ teaspoons salt, divided
1 (15-ounce / 425-g) can diced tomatoes
½ teaspoon freshly ground black pepper

1. Heat the olive oil in a large skillet over medium heat.
2. Add the onion and garlic and sauté for 1 minute until fragrant.
3. Stir in the green beans and sauté for 3 minutes. Sprinkle with ½ teaspoon of salt.
4. Add the tomatoes, remaining salt, and pepper and stir to mix well. Cook for an additional 12 minutes, stirring occasionally, or until the green beans are crisp and tender.
5. Remove from the heat and serve warm.

Tips: To add more flavors to this meal, top the green beans with a sprinkle of toasted pine nuts or almonds before serving. For a spicy kick, you can sprinkle with ½ teaspoon red pepper flakes.

Per Serving
calories: 219 | fat: 13.9g
protein: 4.0g | carbs: 17.7g
fiber: 6.2g | sodium: 843mg

Baked Tomatoes and chickpeas

Prep time: 15 minutes | Cook time: 40 to 45 minutes
Serves 4

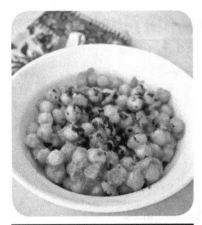

1 tablespoon extra-virgin olive oil
½ medium onion, chopped
3 garlic cloves, chopped
¼ teaspoon ground cumin
2 teaspoons smoked paprika
2 (15-ounce / 425-g) cans chickpeas, drained and rinsed
4 cups halved cherry tomatoes
½ cup plain Greek yogurt, for serving
1 cup crumbled feta cheese, for serving

1. Preheat the oven to 425ºF (220ºC).
2. Heat the olive oil in an ovenproof skillet over medium heat.
3. Add the onion and garlic and sauté for about 5 minutes, stirring occasionally, or until tender and fragrant.
4. Add the paprika and cumin and cook for 2 minutes. Stir in the chickpeas and tomatoes and allow to simmer for 5 to 10 minutes.
5. Transfer the skillet to the preheated oven and roast for 25 to 30 minutes, or until the mixture bubbles and thickens.
6. Remove from the oven and serve topped with yogurt and crumbled feta cheese.

Tips: If you want to make it a vegan dish, you can skip the plain Greek yogurt and feta cheese topping. To add more flavors to this dish, serve the chickpeas and tomatoes over the cauliflower rice or quinoa.

Per Serving
calories: 411 | fat: 14.9g
protein: 20.2g | carbs: 50.7g
fiber: 13.3g | sodium: 443mg

Creamy Cauliflower Chickpea Curry

Prep time: 5 minutes | Cook time: 15 minutes
Serves 4

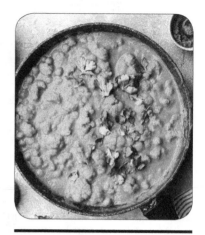

30m or less

3 cups fresh or frozen cauliflower florets
2 cups unsweetened almond milk
1 (15-ounce / 425-g) can low-sodium chickpeas, drained and rinsed
1 (15-ounce / 425-g) can coconut milk
1 tablespoon curry powder
¼ teaspoon garlic powder
¼ teaspoon ground ginger
⅛ teaspoon onion powder
¼ teaspoon salt

1. Add the cauliflower florets, almond milk, chickpeas, coconut milk, curry powder, garlic powder, ginger, and onion powder to a large stockpot and stir to combine.
2. Cover and cook over medium-high heat for 10 minutes, stirring occasionally.
3. Reduce the heat to low and continue cooking uncovered for 5 minutes, or until the cauliflower is tender.
4. Sprinkle with the salt and stir well. Serve warm.

Tip: For added protein, you can serve the curry with a side salad. For added flavor, sprinkle with some chopped fresh cilantro.

Per Serving
calories: 409 | fat: 29.6g
protein: 10.0g | carbs: 29.8g
fiber: 9.1g | sodium: 117mg

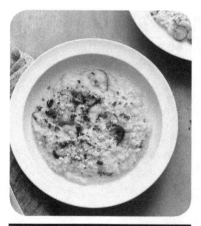

Cauliflower Rice Risotto with Mushrooms

Prep time: 5 minutes | Cook time: 10 minutes
Serves 4

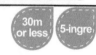

30m or less   5-ingre

1 teaspoon extra-virgin olive oil
½ cup chopped portobello mushrooms
4 cups cauliflower rice
½ cup half-and-half
¼ cup low-sodium vegetable broth
1 cup shredded Parmesan cheese

1. In a medium skillet, heat the olive oil over medium-low heat until shimmering.
2. Add the mushrooms and stir-fry for 3 minutes.
3. Stir in the cauliflower rice, half-and-half, and vegetable broth. Cover and bring to a boil over high heat for 5 minutes, stirring occasionally.
4. Add the Parmesan cheese and stir to combine. Continue cooking for an additional 3 minutes until the cheese is melted.
5. Divide the mixture into four bowls and serve warm.

Tip: This risotto uses the cauliflower rice different from the traditional risotto. The cauliflower rice is low-carb and it saves your cooking time.

Per Serving
calories: 167 | fat: 10.7g
protein: 12.1g | carbs: 8.1g
fiber: 3.0g | sodium: 326mg

Stuffed Portobello Mushrooms with Spinach

Prep time: 5 minutes | Cook time: 20 minutes
Serves 4

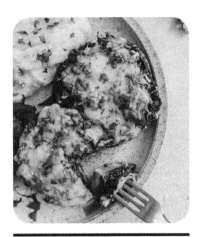

8 large portobello mushrooms, stems removed
3 teaspoons extra-virgin olive oil, divided
1 medium red bell pepper, diced
4 cups fresh spinach
¼ cup crumbled feta cheese

1. Preheat the oven to 450ºF (235ºC).
2. Using a spoon to scoop out the gills of the mushrooms and discard them. Brush the mushrooms with 2 teaspoons of olive oil.
3. Arrange the mushrooms (cap-side down) on a baking sheet. Roast in the preheated oven for 20 minutes.
4. Meantime, in a medium skillet, heat the remaining olive oil over medium heat until it shimmers.
5. Add the bell pepper and spinach and sauté for 8 to 10 minutes, stirring occasionally, or until the spinach is wilted.
6. Remove the mushrooms from the oven to a paper towel-lined plate. Using a spoon to stuff each mushroom with the bell pepper and spinach mixture. Scatter the feta cheese all over.
7. Serve immediately.

Tip: For more bulk and flavor, you can add a green or yellow bell pepper to this filling.

Per Serving (2 mushrooms)
calories: 115 | fat: 5.9g
protein: 7.2g | carbs: 11.5g
fiber: 4.0g | sodium: 125mg

Chickpea Lettuce Wraps with Celery

Prep time: 10 minutes | Cook time: 0 minutes
Serves 4

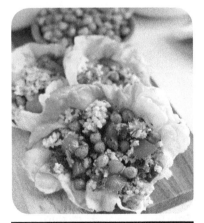

1 (15-ounce / 425-g) can low-sodium chickpeas, drained and rinsed
1 celery stalk, thinly sliced
2 tablespoons finely chopped red onion
2 tablespoons unsalted tahini
3 tablespoons honey mustard
1 tablespoon capers, undrained
12 butter lettuce leaves

1. In a bowl, mash the chickpeas with a potato masher or the back of a fork until mostly smooth.
2. Add the celery, red onion, tahini, honey mustard, and capers to the bowl and stir until well incorporated.
3. For each serving, place three overlapping lettuce leaves on a plate and top with ¼ of the mashed chickpea filling, then roll up. Repeat with the remaining lettuce leaves and chickpea mixture.

Tips: To make this a complete meal, serve the wraps with ¼ cup baby carrots topped with 1 to 2 tablespoon hummus or 1 to 2 hard-boiled eggs. And you can try this recipe with romaine or green leaf lettuce.

Per Serving
calories: 182 | fat: 7.1g
protein: 10.3g | carbs: 19.6g
fiber: 3.0g | sodium: 171mg

Grilled Lemon Chicken

Prep time: 10 minutes | Cook time: 12 to 14 minutes
Serves 2

Marinade:

4 tablespoons freshly squeezed lemon juice
2 tablespoons olive oil, plus more for greasing the grill grates
1 teaspoon dried basil

1 teaspoon paprika
½ teaspoon dried thyme
¼ teaspoon salt
¼ teaspoon garlic powder

2 (4-ounce / 113-g) boneless, skinless chicken breasts

1. Make the marinade: Whisk together the lemon juice, olive oil, basil, paprika, thyme, salt, and garlic powder in a large bowl until well combined.
2. Add the chicken breasts to the bowl and let marinate for at least 30 minutes.
3. When ready to cook, preheat the grill to medium-high heat. Lightly grease the grill grates with the olive oil.
4. Discard the marinade and arrange the chicken breasts on the grill grates.
5. Grill for 12 to 14 minutes, flipping the chicken halfway through, or until a meat thermometer inserted in the center of the chicken reaches 165ºF (74ºC).
6. Let the chicken cool for 5 minutes and serve warm.

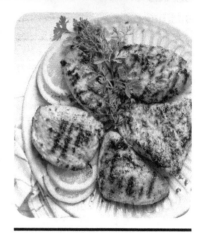

Tip: You can add any of your favorite spices or herbs to this marinade. To make this a complete meal, you can serve it with sautéed green beans and mashed potatoes.

Per Serving

calories: 251 | fat: 15.5g
protein: 27.3g | carbs: 1.9g
fiber: 1.0g | sodium: 371mg

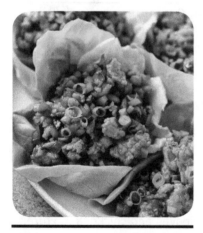

Tips: You can cover the bottom half of each salad wrap in foil, for it's easier to eat. If you cannot find the pita bread, whole-grain naan bread will work, too.

Per Serving

calories: 428 | fat: 10.6g
protein: 31.1g | carbs: 50.9g
fiber: 6.0g | sodium: 675mg

Quick Chicken Salad Wraps

Prep time: 15 minutes | Cook time: 0 minutes
Serves 2

30m or less

Tzatziki Sauce:

½ cup plain Greek yogurt
1 tablespoon freshly squeezed lemon juice
Pinch garlic powder

1 teaspoon dried dill
Salt and freshly ground black pepper, to taste

Salad Wraps:

2 (8-inch) whole-grain pita bread
1 cup shredded chicken meat
2 cups mixed greens
2 roasted red bell peppers, thinly sliced

½ English cucumber, peeled if desired and thinly sliced
¼ cup pitted black olives
1 scallion, chopped

1. Make the tzatziki sauce: In a bowl, whisk together the yogurt, lemon juice, garlic powder, dill, salt, and pepper until creamy and smooth.
2. Make the salad wraps: Place the pita bread on a clean work surface and spoon ¼ cup of the tzatziki sauce onto each piece of pita bread, spreading it all over. Top with the shredded chicken, mixed greens, red pepper slices, cucumber slices, black olives, finished by chopped scallion.
3. Roll the salad wraps and enjoy.

Baked Teriyaki Turkey Meatballs

Prep time: 20 minutes | Cook time: 20 minutes
Serves 6

1 pound (454 g) lean ground turkey
1 egg, whisked
¼ cup finely chopped scallions, both white and green parts
2 garlic cloves, minced
2 tablespoons reduced-sodium tamari or gluten-free soy sauce
1 teaspoon grated fresh ginger
1 tablespoon honey
2 teaspoons mirin
1 teaspoon olive oil

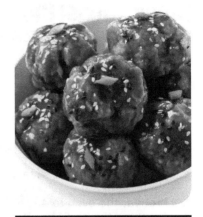

1. Preheat the oven to 400ºF (205ºC). Line a baking sheet with parchment paper and set aside.
2. Mix together the ground turkey, whisked egg, scallions, garlic, tamari, ginger, honey, mirin, and olive oil in a large bowl, and stir until well blended.
3. Using a tablespoon to scoop out rounded heaps of the turkey mixture, and then roll them into balls with your hands. Transfer the balls to the prepared baking sheet.
4. Bake in the preheated oven for 20 minutes, flipping the balls with a spatula halfway through, or until the meatballs are browned and cooked through.
5. Serve warm.

Tip: Teriyaki is a cooking technique used in Japanese cuisine where foods are broiled or grilled with a glaze of soy sauce, mirin, and sugar. In this recipe, the sugar is replaced with honey, and it is still packed with teriyaki flavor.

Per Serving
calories: 158 | fat: 8.6g
protein: 16.2g | carbs: 4.0g
fiber: 0.2g | sodium: 269mg

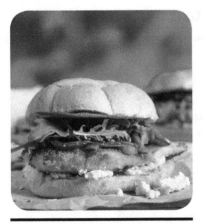

Tip: Use any leftovers to your favorite salad. You can cook the patties in a nonstick skillet over medium-high, 4 to 5 minutes per side, until cooked through.

Per Serving
calories: 241 | fat: 13.5g
protein: 23.2g | carbs:6.7g
fiber: 1.1g | sodium: 321mg

Panko Grilled Chicken Patties

Prep time: 10 minutes | Cook time: 8 to 10 minutes
Serves 4

30m or less

1 pound (454 g) ground chicken
3 tablespoons crumbled feta cheese
3 tablespoons finely chopped red pepper
¼ cup finely chopped red onion
3 tablespoons panko bread crumbs
1 garlic clove, minced
1 teaspoon chopped fresh oregano
¼ teaspoon salt
⅛ teaspoon freshly ground black pepper
Cooking spray

1. Mix together the ground chicken, feta cheese, red pepper, red onion, bread crumbs, garlic, oregano, salt, and black pepper in a large bowl, and stir to incorporate.
2. Divide the chicken mixture into 8 equal portions and form each portion into a patty with your hands.
3. Preheat a grill to medium-high heat and oil the grill grates with cooking spray.
4. Arrange the patties on the grill grates and grill each side for 4 to 5 minutes, or until the patties are cooked through.
5. Rest for 5 minutes before serving.

Spiced Roast Chicken

Prep time: 10 minutes | Cook time: 35 minutes
Serves 6

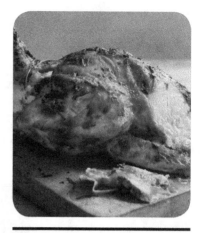

1 teaspoon garlic powder
1 teaspoon ground paprika
½ teaspoon ground cumin
½ teaspoon ground coriander
½ teaspoon salt
¼ teaspoon ground cayenne pepper
6 chicken legs
1 teaspoon extra-virgin olive oil

1. Preheat the oven to 400ºF (205ºC).
2. Combine the garlic powder, paprika, cumin, coriander, salt, and cayenne pepper in a small bowl.
3. On a clean work surface, rub the spices all over the chicken legs until completely coated.
4. Heat the olive oil in an ovenproof skillet over medium heat.
5. Add the chicken thighs and sear each side for 8 to 10 minutes, or until the skin is crispy and browned.
6. Transfer the skillet to the preheated oven and continue cooking for 10 to 15 minutes, or until the juices run clear and it registers an internal temperature of 165ºF (74ºC).
7. Remove from the heat and serve on plates.

Tip: The skin-on, bone-in chicken breasts would work just as well as chicken legs with this spice rub. The chicken breasts take longer to cook. Bake for 45 minutes until cooked through, flipping halfway through.

Per Serving
calories: 275 | fat: 15.6g
protein: 30.3g | carbs: 0.9g
fiber: 0g | sodium: 255mg

Yogurt Chicken Breasts

Prep time: 10 minutes | Cook time: 10 minutes
Serves 4

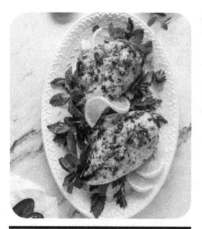

Tips: If the saffron isn't available, you can use ½ teaspoon of turmeric to replace it. To make this a complete meal, serve it with your favorite salad or cooked brown rice.

Per Serving
calories: 154 | fat: 4.8g
protein: 26.3g | carbs: 2.9g
fiber: 0g | sodium: 500mg

Yogurt Sauce:
½ cup plain Greek yogurt
2 tablespoons water
Pinch saffron (3 or 4 threads)
3 garlic cloves, minced
½ onion, chopped
2 tablespoons chopped fresh cilantro
Juice of ½ lemon
½ teaspoon salt

1 pound (454 g) boneless, skinless chicken breasts, cut into 2-inch strips
1 tablespoon extra-virgin olive oil

1. Make the yogurt sauce: Place the yogurt, water, saffron, garlic, onion, cilantro, lemon juice, and salt in a blender, and pulse until completely mixed.
2. Transfer the yogurt sauce to a large bowl, along with the chicken strips. Toss to coat well.
3. Cover with plastic wrap and marinate in the refrigerator for at least 1 hour, or up to overnight.
4. When ready to cook, heat the olive oil in a large skillet over medium heat.
5. Add the chicken strips to the skillet, discarding any excess marinade. Cook each side for 5 minutes, or until cooked through.
6. Let the chicken cool for 5 minutes before serving.

Coconut Chicken Tenders

Prep time: 10 minutes | Cook time: 15 to 20 minutes
Serves 6

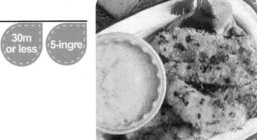

4 chicken breasts, each cut lengthwise into 3 strips
½ teaspoon salt
¼ teaspoon freshly ground black pepper
½ cup coconut flour
2 eggs
2 tablespoons unsweetened plain almond milk
1 cup unsweetened coconut flakes

1. Preheat the oven to 400ºF (205ºC). Line a baking sheet with parchment paper.
2. On a clean work surface, season the chicken with salt and pepper.
3. In a small bowl, add the coconut flour. In a separate bowl, whisk the eggs with almond milk until smooth. Place the coconut flakes on a plate.
4. One at a time, roll the chicken strips in the coconut flour, then dredge them in the egg mixture, shaking off any excess, and finally in the coconut flakes to coat.
5. Arrange the coated chicken pieces on the baking skeet. Bake in the preheated oven for 15 to 20 minutes, flipping the chicken halfway through, or until the chicken is golden brown and cooked through.
6. Remove from the oven and serve on plates.

Tip: The chicken tenders can be served with anything you like. They taste great with a small potato with a green salad.

Per Serving
calories: 215 | fat: 12.6g
protein: 20.2g | carbs: 8.9g
fiber: 6.1g | sodium: 345mg

Sautéed Ground Turkey with Brown Rice

Prep time: 20 minutes | Cook time: 45 minutes
Serves 2

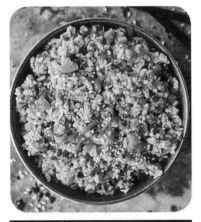

1 tablespoon olive oil
½ medium onion, minced
2 garlic cloves, minced
8 ounces (227 g) ground turkey breast
½ cup chopped roasted red peppers, (about 2 jarred peppers)
¼ cup sun-dried tomatoes, minced
1¼ cups low-sodium chicken stock
½ cup brown rice
1 teaspoon dried oregano
Salt, to taste
2 cups lightly packed baby spinach

Per Serving
calories: 445 | fat: 16.8g
protein: 30.2g | carbs: 48.9g
fiber: 5.1g | sodium: 662mg

1. In a skillet, heat the olive oil over medium heat. Sauté the onion for 5 minutes, stirring occasionally.
2. Stir in the garlic and sauté for 30 seconds more until fragrant.
3. Add the turkey breast and cook for about 7 minutes, breaking apart with a wooden spoon, until the turkey is no longer pink.
4. Stir in the roasted red peppers, tomatoes, chicken stock, brown rice, and oregano and bring to a boil.
5. When the mixture starts to boil, cover, and reduce the heat to medium-low. Bring to a simmer until the rice is tender, stirring occasionally, about 30 minutes. Sprinkle with the salt.
6. Add the baby spinach and keep stirring until wilted.
7. Remove from the heat and serve warm.

Lamb Tagine with Couscous and Almonds

Prep time: 15 minutes | Cook time: 7 hours 7 minutes
Serves 6

2 tablespoons almond flour
Juice and zest of 1 navel orange
2 tablespoons extra-virgin olive oil
2 pounds (907 g) boneless lamb leg, fat trimmed and cut into 1½-inch cubes
½ cup low-sodium chicken stock
2 large white onions, chopped
1 teaspoon pumpkin pie spice
¼ teaspoon crushed saffron threads
1 teaspoon ground cumin
¼ teaspoon ground red pepper flakes
½ teaspoon sea salt
2 tablespoons raw honey
1 cup pitted dates
3 cups cooked couscous, for serving
2 tablespoons toasted slivered almonds, for serving

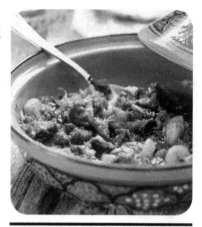

1. Combine the almond flour with orange juice in a large bowl. Stir until smooth, then mix in the orange zest. Set aside.
2. Heat the olive oil in a nonstick skillet over medium-high heat until shimmering.
3. Add the lamb cubes and sauté for 7 minutes or until lightly browned.
4. Pour in the flour mixture and chicken stock, then add the onions, pumpkin pie spice, saffron, cumin, ground red pepper flakes, and salt. Stir to mix well.
5. Pour them in the slow cooker. Cover and cook on low for 6 hours or until the internal temperature of the lamb reaches at least 145ºF (63ºC).
6. When the cooking is complete, mix in the honey and dates, then cook for another an hour.
7. Put the couscous in a tagine bowl or a simple large bowl, then top with lamb mixture. Scatter with slivered almonds and serve immediately.

Tip: How to cook the couscous: Bring a saucepan of salted water to a boil. Turn off the heat, then add the couscous and cover the pan. Stream the couscous for 5 minutes or until tender. Fluff with a fork.

Per Serving
calories: 447 | fat: 10.2g
protein: 36.3g | carbs: 53.5g
fiber: 4.9g | sodium: 329mg

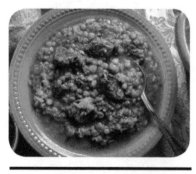

Beef, Tomato, and Lentils Stew

Prep time: 10 minutes | Cook time: 10 minutes
Serves 4

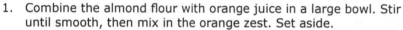

1 tablespoon extra-virgin olive oil
1 pound (454 g) extra-lean ground beef
1 onion, chopped
1 (14-ounce / 397-g) can chopped tomatoes with garlic and basil, drained
1 (14-ounce / 397-g) can lentils, drained
½ teaspoon sea salt
⅛ teaspoon freshly ground black pepper

Tip: If you want to remove as much salt that contains in the canned beans as possible, drain the canned beans in a colander and rinse under running cold water, then pat dry with paper towels.

1. Heat the olive oil in a pot over medium-high heat until shimmering.
2. Add the beef and onion to the pot and sauté for 5 minutes or until the beef is lightly browned.
3. Add the remaining ingredients. Bring to a boil. Reduce the heat to medium and cook for 4 more minutes or until the lentils are tender. Keep stirring during the cooking.
4. Pour them in a large serving bowl and serve immediately.

Per Serving
calories: 460 | fat: 14.8g
protein: 44.2g | carbs: 36.9g
fiber: 17.0g | sodium: 320mg

Herbed-Mustard-Coated Pork Tenderloin

Prep time: 10 minutes | Cook time: 15 minutes
Serves 4

3 tablespoons fresh rosemary leaves
¼ cup Dijon mustard
½ cup fresh parsley leaves
6 garlic cloves
½ teaspoon sea salt
¼ teaspoon freshly ground black pepper
1 tablespoon extra-virgin olive oil
1 (1½-pound / 680-g) pork tenderloin

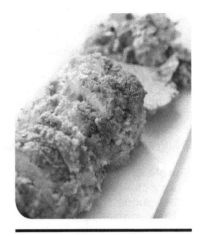

1. Preheat the oven to 400ºF (205ºC).
2. Put all the ingredients, except for the pork tenderloin, in a food processor. Pulse until it has a thick consistency.
3. Put the pork tenderloin on a baking sheet, then rub with the mixture to coat well.
4. Put the sheet in the preheated oven and bake for 15 minutes or until the internal temperature of the pork reaches at least 165ºF (74ºC). Flip the tenderloin halfway through the cooking time.
5. Transfer the cooked pork tenderloin to a large plate and allow to cool for 5 minutes before serving.

Tip: If you want to make your pork hotter, you can add a touch of crushed jalapeño to the mixture in the food processor.

Per Serving
calories: 363 | fat: 18.1g
protein: 2.2g | carbs: 4.9g
fiber: 2.0g | sodium: 514mg

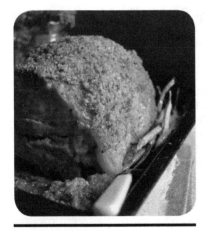

Tip: To make this a complete meal, you can serve it with roasted cauliflower. Or you can use it as a snack to serve during the brunch time. Or you can use it as the filling to make the burgers.

Per Serving
calories: 436 | fat: 32.8g
protein: 33.1g | carbs: 5.9g
fiber: 3.0g | sodium: 310mg

Macadamia Pork

Prep time: 10 minutes | Cook time: 10 minutes
Serves 4

30m or less *5-ingre*

1 (1-pound / 454-g) pork tenderloin, cut into ½-inch slices and pounded thin
1 teaspoon sea salt, divided
¼ teaspoon freshly ground black

pepper, divided
½ cup macadamia nuts
1 cup unsweetened coconut milk
1 tablespoon extra-virgin olive oil

1. Preheat the oven to 400ºF (205ºC).
2. On a clean work surface, rub the pork with ½ teaspoon of the salt and ⅛ teaspoon of the ground black pepper. Set aside.
3. Ground the macadamia nuts in a food processor, then combine with remaining salt and black pepper in a bowl. Stir to mix well and set aside.
4. Combine the coconut milk and olive oil in a separate bowl. Stir to mix well.
5. Dredge the pork chops into the bowl of coconut milk mixture, then dunk into the bowl of macadamia nut mixture to coat well. Shake the excess off.
6. Put the well-coated pork chops on a baking sheet, then bake for 10 minutes or until the internal temperature of the pork reaches at least 165ºF (74ºC).
7. Transfer the pork chops to a serving plate and serve immediately.

Ground Beef, Tomato, and Kidney Bean Chili

Prep time: 10 minutes | Cook time: 15 minutes
Serves 4

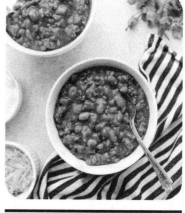

1 tablespoon extra-virgin olive oil
1 pound (454 g) extra-lean ground beef
1 onion, chopped
2 (14-ounce / 397-g) cans kidney beans
2 (28-ounce / 794-g) cans chopped tomatoes, juice reserved

Simple Chili Spice:
1 teaspoon garlic powder
1 tablespoon chili powder
½ teaspoon sea salt

1. Heat the olive oil in a pot over medium-high heat until shimmering.
2. Add the beef and onion to the pot and sauté for 5 minutes or until the beef is lightly browned and the onion is translucent.
3. Add the remaining ingredients. Bring to a boil. Reduce the heat to medium and cook for 10 more minutes. Keep stirring during the cooking.
4. Pour them in a large serving bowl and serve immediately.

Tip: You can make your own chili spice for this recipe by mixing chili powder, dried oregano, onion powder, cumin, garlic powder, ground coriander, and sea salt in a 4:2:1:1:1:1:1 ratio.

Per Serving
calories: 891 | fat: 20.1g
protein: 116.3g | carbs: 62.9g
fiber: 17.0g | sodium: 561mg

Slow Cook Lamb Shanks with Cannellini Beans Stew

Prep time: 20 minutes | Cook time: 10 hours 15 minutes
Serves 12

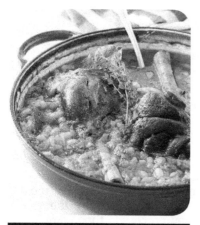

1 (19-ounce / 539-g) can cannellini beans, rinsed and drained
1 large yellow onion, chopped
2 medium-sized carrots, diced
1 large stalk celery, chopped
2 cloves garlic, thinly sliced

4 (1½-pound / 680-g) lamb shanks, fat trimmed
2 teaspoons tarragon
½ teaspoon sea salt
¼ teaspoon ground black pepper
1 (28-ounce / 794-g) can diced tomatoes, with the juice

1. Combine the beans, onion, carrots, celery, and garlic in the slow cooker. Stir to mix well.
2. Add the lamb shanks and sprinkle with tarragon, salt, and ground black pepper.
3. Pour in the tomatoes with juice, then cover the lid and cook on high for an hour.
4. Reduce the heat to low and cook for 9 hours or until the lamb is super tender.
5. Transfer the lamb on a plate, then pour the bean mixture in a colander over a separate bowl to reserve the liquid.
6. Let the liquid sit for 5 minutes until set, then skim the fat from the surface of the liquid. Pour the bean mixture back to the liquid.
7. Remove the bones from the lamb heat and discard the bones. Put the lamb meat and bean mixture back to the slow cooker. Cover and cook to reheat for 15 minutes or until heated through.
8. Pour them on a large serving plate and serve immediately.

Tip: If you want to remove as much salt that contains in the canned beans as possible, drain the canned beans in a colander and rinse under running cold water, then pat dry with paper towels.

Per Serving
calories: 317 | fat: 9.7g
protein: 52.1g | carbs: 7.0g
fiber: 2.1g | sodium: 375mg

Potato Lamb and Olive Stew

Prep time: 20 minutes | Cook time: 3 hours 42 minutes
Serves 10

4 tablespoons almond flour
¾ cup low-sodium chicken stock
1¼ pounds (567 g) small potatoes, halved
3 cloves garlic, minced
4 large shallots, cut into ½-inch wedges
3 sprigs fresh rosemary
1 tablespoon lemon zest
Coarse sea salt and black pepper, to taste
3½ pounds (1.6 kg) lamb shanks, fat trimmed and cut crosswise into 1½-inch pieces
2 tablespoons extra-virgin olive oil
½ cup dry white wine
1 cup pitted green olives, halved
2 tablespoons lemon juice

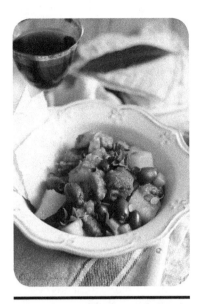

1. Combine 1 tablespoon of almond flour with chicken stock in a bowl. Stir to mix well.
2. Put the flour mixture, potatoes, garlic, shallots, rosemary, and lemon zest in the slow cooker. Sprinkle with salt and black pepper. Stir to mix well. Set aside.
3. Combine the remaining almond flour with salt and black pepper in a large bowl, then dunk the lamb shanks in the flour and toss to coat.
4. Heat the olive oil in a nonstick skillet over medium-high heat until shimmering.
5. Add the well-coated lamb and cook for 10 minutes or until golden brown. Flip the lamb pieces halfway through the cooking time. Transfer the cooked lamb to the slow cooker.
6. Pour the wine in the same skillet, then cook for 2 minutes or until it reduces in half. Pour the wine in the slow cooker.
7. Put the slow cooker lid on and cook on high for 3 hours and 30 minutes or until the lamb is very tender.
8. In the last 20 minutes of the cooking, open the lid and fold in the olive halves to cook.
9. Pour the stew on a large plate, let them sit for 5 minutes, then skim any fat remains over the face of the liquid.
10. Drizzle with lemon juice and sprinkle with salt and pepper. Serve warm.

Tip: To make this a complete meal, you can serve it with roasted root vegetables and mushroom soup.

Per Serving
calories: 309 | fat: 10.3g
protein: 36.9g | carbs: 16.1g
fiber: 2.2g | sodium: 239mg

Roasted Chicken Thighs With Basmati Rice

Prep time: 15 minutes | Cook time: 50 to 55 minutes
Serves 2

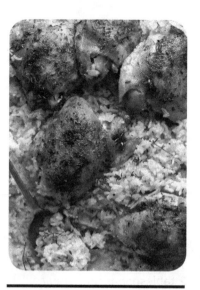

Chicken:
½ teaspoon cumin
½ teaspoon cinnamon
½ teaspoon paprika
¼ teaspoon ginger powder
¼ teaspoon garlic powder
¼ teaspoon coriander
¼ teaspoon salt
⅛ teaspoon cayenne pepper
10 ounces (284 g) boneless, skinless chicken thighs (about 4 pieces)

Rice:
1 tablespoon olive oil
½ small onion, minced
½ cup basmati rice
2 pinches saffron
1 cup low-sodium chicken stock
¼ teaspoon salt

Tip: You can substitute the boneless or bone-in chicken breasts for chicken thighs.

Per Serving
calories: 400 | fat: 9.6g
protein: 37.2g | carbs: 40.7g
fiber: 2.1g | sodium: 714mg

Make the Chicken
1. Preheat the oven to 350ºF (180ºC).
2. Combine the cumin, cinnamon, paprika, ginger powder, garlic powder, coriander, salt, and cayenne pepper in a small bowl.
3. Using your hands to rub the spice mixture all over the chicken thighs.
4. Transfer the chicken thighs to a baking dish. Roast in the preheated oven for 35 to 40 minutes, or until the internal temperature reaches 165ºF (74ºC) on a meat thermometer.

Make the Rice
1. Meanwhile, heat the olive oil in a skillet over medium-high heat.
2. Sauté the onion for 5 minutes until fragrant, stirring occasionally.
3. Stir in the basmati rice, saffron, chicken stock, and salt. Reduce the heat to low, cover, and bring to a simmer for 15 minutes, until light and fluffy.
4. Remove the chicken from the oven to a plate and serve with the rice.

Chapter 9 Fish and Seafood

Air-Fried Flounder Fillets

Prep time: 5 minutes | Cook time: 12 minutes
Serves 4

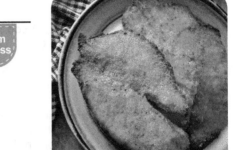

2 cups unsweetened almond milk
½ teaspoon onion powder
½ teaspoon garlic powder
4 (4-ounce / 113-g) flounder fillets
½ cup chickpea flour
½ cup plain yellow cornmeal
¼ teaspoon cayenne pepper
Freshly ground black pepper, to taste

1. Whisk together the almond milk, onion powder, and garlic powder in a large bowl until smooth.
2. Add the flounder, coating well on both sides, and let marinate for about 20 minutes.
3. Meanwhile, combine the chickpea flour, cornmeal, cayenne, and pepper in a shallow dish.
4. Dredge each piece of flounder fillets in the flour mixture until completely coated.
5. Preheat the air fryer to 380ºF (193ºC).
6. Arrange the coated flounder fillets in the basket and cook for 12 minutes, flipping them halfway through.
7. Remove from the basket and serve on a plate.

Tip: If an air fryer isn't available, you can place the flounder fillets on a rimmed baking sheet and broil for 12 minutes, flipping once halfway through.

Per Serving
calories: 228 | fat: 5.7g
protein: 28.2g | carbs: 15.5g
fiber: 2.0g | sodium: 240mg

10-Minute Cod with Parsley Pistou

Prep time: 15 minutes | Cook time: 10 minutes
Serves 4

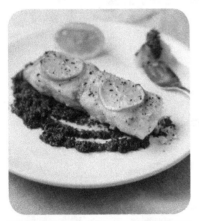

1 cup packed roughly chopped fresh flat-leaf Italian parsley
Zest and juice of 1 lemon
1 to 2 small garlic cloves, minced
1 teaspoon salt
½ teaspoon freshly ground black pepper
1 cup extra-virgin olive oil, divided
1 pound (454 g) cod fillets, cut into 4 equal-sized pieces

1. Make the pistou: Place the parsley, lemon zest and juice, garlic, salt, and pepper in a food processor until finely chopped.
2. With the food processor running, slowly drizzle in ¾ cup of olive oil until a thick sauce forms. Set aside.
3. Heat the remaining ¼ cup of olive oil in a large skillet over medium-high heat.
4. Add the cod fillets, cover, and cook each side for 4 to 5 minutes, until browned and cooked through.
5. Remove the cod fillets from the heat to a plate and top each with generous spoonfuls of the prepared pistou. Serve immediately.

Tip: You can serve the pistou on steamed vegetables, toasted whole-wheat bread, salads, and other grilled meats or seafoods.

Per Serving
calories: 580 | fat: 54.6g
protein: 21.1g | carbs: 2.8g
fiber: 1.0g | sodium: 651mg

Simple Fried Cod Fillets

Prep time: 5 minutes | Cook time: 10 minutes
Serves 4

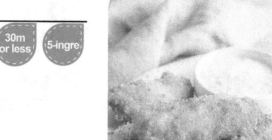

½ cup all-purpose flour
1 teaspoon garlic powder
1 teaspoon salt
4 (4- to 5-ounce / 113- to 142-g) cod fillets
1 tablespoon extra-virgin olive oil

1. Mix together the flour, garlic powder, and salt in a shallow dish.
2. Dredge each piece of fish in the seasoned flour until they are evenly coated.
3. Heat the olive oil in a medium skillet over medium-high heat.
4. Once hot, add the cod fillets and fry for 6 to 8 minutes, flipping the fish halfway through, or until the fish is opaque and flakes easily.
5. Remove from the heat and serve on plates.

Tip: You can use any variety of spices or herbs to season the flour, such as onion powder, paprika, black pepper, oregano, marjoram, or even tarragon.

Per Serving
calories: 333 | fat: 18.8g
protein: 21.2g | carbs: 20.0g
fiber: 5.7g | sodium: 870mg

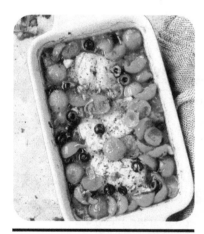

Tip: The cod can be substituted with other lean white fish such as bass, tilapia, haddock and halibut.

Per Serving
calories: 332 | fat: 10.5g
protein: 29.2g | carbs: 30.7g
fiber: 8.0g | sodium: 1906mg

Mediterranean Braised Cod with Vegetables

Prep time: 10 minutes | Cook time: 18 minutes
Serves 2

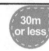

1 tablespoon olive oil
½ medium onion, minced
2 garlic cloves, minced
1 teaspoon oregano
1 (15-ounce / 425-g) can artichoke hearts in water, drained and halved
1 (15-ounce / 425-g) can diced tomatoes with basil
¼ cup pitted Greek olives, drained
10 ounces (284 g) wild cod
Salt and freshly ground black pepper, to taste

1. In a skillet, heat the olive oil over medium-high heat.
2. Sauté the onion for about 5 minutes, stirring occasionally, or until tender.
3. Stir in the garlic and oregano and cook for 30 seconds more until fragrant.
4. Add the artichoke hearts, tomatoes, and olives and stir to combine. Top with the cod.
5. Cover and cook for 10 minutes, or until the fish flakes easily with a fork and juices run clean.
6. Sprinkle with the salt and pepper. Serve warm.

Lemon-Parsley Swordfish

Prep time: 10 minutes | Cook time: 17 to 20 minutes
Serves 4

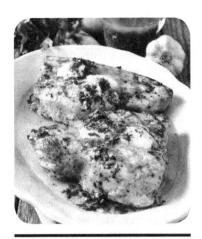

1 cup fresh Italian parsley
¼ cup lemon juice
¼ cup extra-virgin olive oil
¼ cup fresh thyme
2 cloves garlic
½ teaspoon salt
4 swordfish steaks
Olive oil spray

1. Preheat the oven to 450ºF (235ºC). Grease a large baking dish generously with olive oil spray.
2. Place the parsley, lemon juice, olive oil, thyme, garlic, and salt in a food processor and pulse until smoothly blended.
3. Arrange the swordfish steaks in the greased baking dish and spoon the parsley mixture over the top.
4. Bake in the preheated oven for 17 to 20 minutes until flaky.
5. Divide the fish among four plates and serve hot.

Tips: If you prefer a milder flavor, you can substitute the fresh cilantro or basil for parsley. To make this a complete meal, serve it with a cherry tomato salad.

Per Serving
calories: 396 | fat: 21.7g
protein: 44.2g | carbs: 2.9g
fiber: 1.0g | sodium: 494mg

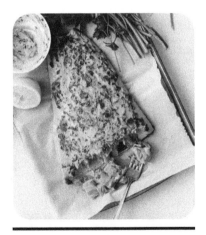

Tip: You can use 1 to 2 teaspoons dried tarragon to replace the fresh tarragon.

Per Serving
calories: 386 | fat: 27.7g
protein: 29.3g | carbs: 3.8g
fiber: 1.0g | sodium: 632mg

Baked Salmon with Tarragon Mustard Sauce

Prep time: 5 minutes | Cook time: 12 minutes
Serves 4

1¼ pounds (567 g) salmon fillet (skin on or removed), cut into 4 equal pieces
¼ cup Dijon mustard
¼ cup avocado oil mayonnaise
Zest and juice of ½ lemon
2 tablespoons chopped fresh tarragon
½ teaspoon salt
¼ teaspoon freshly ground black pepper
4 tablespoons extra-virgin olive oil, for serving

1. Preheat the oven to 425ºF (220ºC). Line a baking sheet with parchment paper.
2. Arrange the salmon pieces on the prepared baking sheet, skin-side down.
3. Stir together the mustard, avocado oil mayonnaise, lemon zest and juice, tarragon, salt, and pepper in a small bowl. Spoon the mustard mixture over the salmon.
4. Bake for 10 to 12 minutes, or until the top is golden and salmon is opaque in the center.
5. Divide the salmon among four plates and drizzle each top with 1 tablespoon of olive oil before serving.

Baked Lemon Salmon

Prep time: 5 minutes | Cook time: 20 minutes
Serves 4

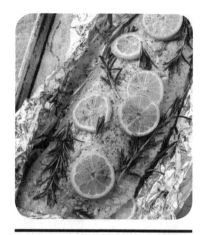

¼ teaspoon dried thyme
Zest and juice of ½ lemon
¼ teaspoon salt
½ teaspoon freshly ground black pepper
1 pound (454 g) salmon fillet
Nonstick cooking spray

1. Preheat the oven to 425°F (220°C). Coat a baking sheet with nonstick cooking spray.
2. Mix together the thyme, lemon zest and juice, salt, and pepper in a small bowl and stir to incorporate.
3. Arrange the salmon, skin-side down, on the coated baking sheet. Spoon the thyme mixture over the salmon and spread it all over.
4. Bake in the preheated oven for about 15 to 20 minutes, or until the fish flakes apart easily. Serve warm.

Tip: To make this a complete meal, you can toss the cut-up asparagus, cauliflower, and broccoli with 1 teaspoon olive oil in a large bowl until well coated and add them to the baking sheet.

Per Serving
calories: 162 | fat: 7.0g
protein: 23.1g | carbs: 1.0g
fiber: 0g | sodium: 166mg

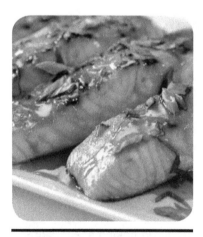

Glazed Broiled Salmon

Prep time: 5 minutes | Cook time: 5 to 10 minutes
Serves 4

4 (4-ounce / 113-g) salmon fillets
3 tablespoons miso paste
2 tablespoons raw honey
1 teaspoon coconut aminos
1 teaspoon rice vinegar

1. Preheat the broiler to High. Line a baking dish with aluminum foil and add the salmon fillets.
2. Whisk together the miso paste, honey, coconut aminos, and vinegar in a small bowl. Pour the glaze over the fillets and spread it evenly with a brush.
3. Broil for about 5 minutes, or until the salmon is browned on top and opaque. Brush any remaining glaze over the salmon and broil for an additional 5 minutes if needed. The cooking time depends on the thickness of the salmon.
4. Let the salmon cool for 5 minutes before serving.

Tip: To add more flavors to this meal, serve the salmon with grilled asparagus or a green salad.

Per Serving
calories: 263 | fat: 8.9g
protein: 30.2g | carbs: 12.8g
fiber: 0.7g | sodium: 716mg

Baked Salmon with Basil and Tomato

Prep time: 10 minutes | Cook time: 20 minutes
Serves 2

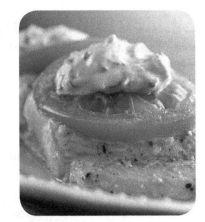

2 (6-ounce / 170-g) boneless salmon fillets
1 tablespoon dried basil
1 tomato, thinly sliced
1 tablespoon olive oil
2 tablespoons grated Parmesan cheese
Nonstick cooking spray

1. Preheat the oven to 375ºF (190ºC). Line a baking sheet with a piece of aluminum foil and mist with nonstick cooking spray.
2. Arrange the salmon fillets onto the aluminum foil and scatter with basil. Place the tomato slices on top and drizzle with olive oil. Top with the grated Parmesan cheese.
3. Bake for about 20 minutes, or until the flesh is opaque and it flakes apart easily.
4. Remove from the oven and serve on a plate.

Per Serving
calories: 403 | fat: 26.5g
protein: 36.3g | carbs: 3.8g
fiber: 0.1g | sodium: 179mg

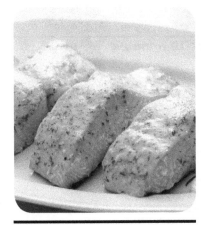

Tip: If the whole-grain mustard isn't available, the Dijon mustard will work, too.

Per Serving
calories: 185 | fat: 7.0g
protein: 23.2g | carbs: 5.8g
fiber: 0g | sodium: 311mg

Honey-Mustard Roasted Salmon

Prep time: 5 minutes | Cook time: 15 to 20 minutes
Serves 4

2 tablespoons whole-grain mustard
2 garlic cloves, minced
1 tablespoon honey
¼ teaspoon salt
¼ teaspoon freshly ground black pepper
1 pound (454 g) salmon fillet
Nonstick cooking spray

1. Preheat the oven to 425ºF (220ºC). Coat a baking sheet with nonstick cooking spray.
2. Stir together the mustard, garlic, honey, salt, and pepper in a small bowl.
3. Arrange the salmon fillet, skin-side down, on the coated baking sheet. Spread the mustard mixture evenly over the salmon fillet.
4. Roast in the preheated oven for 15 to 20 minutes, or until it flakes apart easily and reaches an internal temperature of 145ºF (63ºC).
5. Serve hot.

Salmon and Mushroom Hash with Pesto

Prep time: 15 minutes | Cook time: 20 minutes
Serves 6

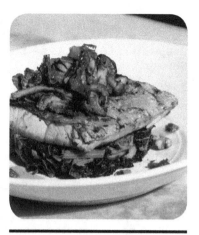

Pesto:
¼ cup extra-virgin olive oil
1 bunch fresh basil
Juice and zest of 1 lemon
1/3 cup water
¼ teaspoon salt, plus additional as needed

Hash:
2 tablespoons extra-virgin olive oil
6 cups mixed mushrooms (brown, white, shiitake, cremini, portobello, etc.), sliced
1 pound (454 g) wild salmon, cubed

1. Make the pesto: Pulse the olive oil, basil, juice and zest, water, and salt in a blender or food processor until smoothly blended. Set aside.
2. Heat the olive oil in a large skillet over medium heat.
3. Stir-fry the mushrooms for 6 to 8 minutes, or until they begin to exude their juices.
4. Add the salmon and cook each side for 5 to 6 minutes until cooked through.
5. Fold in the prepared pesto and stir well. Taste and add additional salt as needed. Serve warm.

Tip: You can use the coconut oil to replace the extra-virgin olive oil.

Per Serving
calories: 264 | fat: 14.7g
protein: 7.0g | carbs: 30.9g
fiber: 4.0g | sodium: 480mg

Spiced Citrus Sole

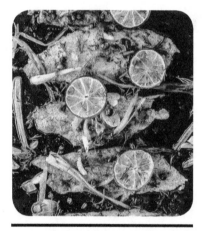

Prep time: 10 minutes | Cook time: 10 minutes
Serves 4

1 teaspoon garlic powder
1 teaspoon chili powder
½ teaspoon lemon zest
½ teaspoon lime zest
¼ teaspoon smoked paprika
¼ teaspoon freshly ground black pepper
Pinch sea salt
4 (6-ounce / 170-g) sole fillets, patted dry
1 tablespoon extra-virgin olive oil
2 teaspoons freshly squeezed lime juice

1. Preheat the oven to 450°F (235°C). Line a baking sheet with aluminum foil and set aside.
2. Mix together the garlic powder, chili powder, lemon zest, lime zest, paprika, pepper, and salt in a small bowl until well combined.
3. Arrange the sole fillets on the prepared baking sheet and rub the spice mixture all over the fillets until well coated. Drizzle the olive oil and lime juice over the fillets.
4. Bake in the preheated oven for about 8 minutes until flaky.
5. Remove from the heat to a plate and serve.

Tip: You can store the spice mixture in an airtight container for up to 2 weeks.

Per Serving
calories: 183 | fat: 5.0g
protein: 32.1g | carbs: 0g
fiber: 0g | sodium: 136mg

Asian-Inspired Tuna Lettuce Wraps

Prep time: 10 minutes | Cook time: 0 minutes
Serves 2

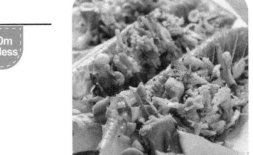

1/3 cup almond butter
1 tablespoon freshly squeezed lemon juice
1 teaspoon low-sodium soy sauce
1 teaspoon curry powder
½ teaspoon sriracha, or to taste
½ cup canned water chestnuts, drained and chopped
2 (2.6-ounce / 74-g) package tuna packed in water, drained
2 large butter lettuce leaves

1. Stir together the almond butter, lemon juice, soy sauce, curry powder, sriracha in a medium bowl until well mixed. Add the water chestnuts and tuna and stir until well incorporated.
2. Place 2 butter lettuce leaves on a flat work surface, spoon half of the tuna mixture onto each leaf and roll up into a wrap. Serve immediately.

Tips: To make this a complete meal, you can serve it with any whole-wheat bread or crackers. You also can spoon the tuna mixture into avocado halves.

Per Serving
calories: 270 | fat: 13.9g
protein: 19.1g | carbs: 18.5g
fiber: 3.0g | sodium: 626mg

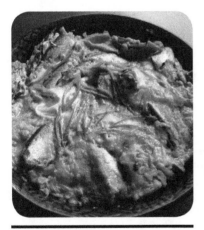

Tips: If you want to save time, you can substitute the quinoa or buckwheat for the brown rice. And the sesame oil can be replaced with extra-virgin olive oil, if desired.

Per Serving
calories: 603 | fat: 23.6g
protein: 25.2g | carbs: 73.8g
fiber: 4.0g | sodium: 498mg

Canned Sardine Donburi (Rice Bowl)

Prep time: 10 minutes | Cook time: 40 to 50 minutes
Serves 4 to 6

4 cups water
2 cups brown rice, rinsed well
½ teaspoon salt
3 (4-ounce / 113-g) cans sardines packed in water, drained
3 scallions, sliced thin
1-inch piece fresh ginger, grated
4 tablespoons sesame oil

1. Place the water, brown rice, and salt to a large saucepan and stir to combine. Allow the mixture to boil over high heat.
2. Once boiling, reduce the heat to low, and cook covered for 45 to 50 minutes, or until the rice is tender.
3. Meanwhile, roughly mash the sardines with a fork in a medium bowl.
4. When the rice is done, stir in the mashed sardines, scallions, and ginger.
5. Divide the mixture into four bowls. Top each bowl with a drizzle of sesame oil. Serve warm.

Spicy Grilled Shrimp with Lemon Wedges

Prep time: 15 minutes | Cook time: 6 minutes
Serves 6

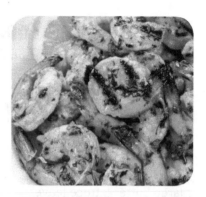

1 large clove garlic, crushed
1 teaspoon coarse salt
1 teaspoon paprika
½ teaspoon cayenne pepper
2 teaspoons lemon juice

2 tablespoons plus 1 teaspoon olive oil, divided
2 pounds (907 g) large shrimp, peeled and deveined
8 wedges lemon, for garnish

1. Preheat the grill to medium heat.
2. Stir together the garlic, salt, paprika, cayenne pepper, lemon juice, and 2 tablespoons of olive oil in a small bowl until a paste forms. Add the shrimp and toss until well coated.
3. Grease the grill grates lightly with remaining 1 teaspoon of olive oil.
4. Grill the shrimp for 4 to 6 minutes, flipping the shrimp halfway through, or until the shrimp is totally pink and opaque.
5. Garnish the shrimp with lemon wedges and serve hot.

Tip: To make this a complete meal, you can serve it with zucchini noodle salad.

Per Serving
calories: 163 | fat: 5.8g
protein: 25.2g | carbs: 2.8g
fiber: 0.4g | sodium: 585mg

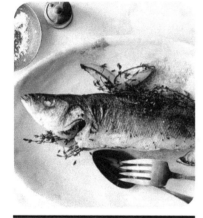

Tip: If you have any leftovers, you can serve with steamed brown rice or roasted potatoes.

Per Serving
calories: 1059 | fat: 71.9g
protein: 46.2g | carbs: 55.8g
fiber: 5.1g | sodium: 2807mg

Braised Branzino with Wine Sauce

Prep time: 15 minutes | Cook time: 15 minutes
Serves 2 to 3

Sauce:
¾ cup dry white wine
2 tablespoons white wine vinegar

2 tablespoons cornstarch
1 tablespoon honey

Fish:
1 large branzino, butterflied and patted dry
2 tablespoons onion powder
2 tablespoons paprika
½ tablespoon salt
6 tablespoons extra-virgin olive oil, divided

4 garlic cloves, thinly sliced
4 scallions, both green and white parts, thinly sliced
1 large tomato, cut into ¼-inch cubes
4 kalamata olives, pitted and chopped

1. Make the sauce: Mix together the white wine, vinegar, cornstarch, and honey in a bowl and keep stirring until the honey has dissolved. Set aside.
2. Make the fish: Place the fish on a clean work surface, skin-side down. Sprinkle the onion powder, paprika, and salt to season. Drizzle 2 tablespoons of olive oil all over the fish.
3. Heat 2 tablespoons of olive oil in a large skillet over high heat until it shimmers.
4. Add the fish, skin-side up, to the skillet and brown for about 2 minutes. Carefully flip the fish and cook for another 3 minutes. Remove from the heat to a plate and set aside.
5. Add the remaining 2 tablespoons olive oil to the skillet and swirl to coat. Stir in the garlic cloves, scallions, tomato, and kalamata olives and sauté for 5 minutes. Pour in the prepared sauce and stir to combine.
6. Return the fish (skin-side down) to the skillet, flipping to coat in the sauce. Reduce the heat to medium-low, and cook for an additional 5 minutes until cooked through.
7. Using a slotted spoon, transfer the fish to a plate and serve warm.

Peppercorn-Seared Tuna Steaks

Prep time: 5 minutes | Cook time: 10 minutes
Serves 2

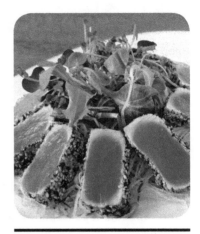

2 (5-ounce / 142-g) ahi tuna steaks
1 teaspoon kosher salt
¼ teaspoon cayenne pepper
2 tablespoons olive oil
1 teaspoon whole peppercorns

1. On a plate, Season the tuna steaks on both sides with salt and cayenne pepper.
2. In a skillet, heat the olive oil over medium-high heat until it shimmers.
3. Add the peppercorns and cook for about 5 minutes, or until they soften and pop.
4. Carefully put the tuna steaks in the skillet and sear for 1 to 2 minutes per side, depending on the thickness of the tuna steaks, or until the fish is cooked to the desired level of doneness.
5. Cool for 5 minutes before serving.

Tip: The seared tuna steaks pair perfectly with crispy green beans or roasted lemon potatoes.

Per Serving
calories: 260 | fat: 14.3g
protein: 33.4g | carbs: 0.2g
fiber: 0.1g | sodium: 1033mg

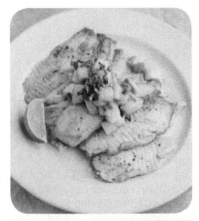

Tip: You can serve the fillets with the pineapple salsa on top. Simple use the same amount of fresh or canned pineapple to replace the mango.

Per Serving
calories: 239 | fat: 7.8g
protein: 25.0g | carbs: 21.9g
fiber: 4.0g | sodium: 416mg

Crispy Tilapia with Mango Salsa

Prep time: 5 minutes | Cook time: 10 minutes
Serves 2

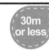

Salsa:
1 cup chopped mango
2 tablespoons chopped fresh cilantro
2 tablespoons chopped red onion
2 tablespoons freshly squeezed
lime juice
½ jalapeño pepper, seeded and minced
Pinch salt

Tilapia:
1 tablespoon paprika
1 teaspoon onion powder
½ teaspoon dried thyme
½ teaspoon freshly ground black pepper
¼ teaspoon cayenne pepper
½ teaspoon garlic powder
¼ teaspoon salt
½ pound (227 g) boneless tilapia fillets
2 teaspoons extra-virgin olive oil
1 lime, cut into wedges, for serving

1. Make the salsa: Place the mango, cilantro, onion, lime juice, jalapeño, and salt in a medium bowl and toss to combine. Set aside.
2. Make the tilapia: Stir together the paprika, onion powder, thyme, black pepper, cayenne pepper, garlic powder, and salt in a small bowl until well mixed. Rub both sides of fillets generously with the mixture.
3. Heat the olive oil in a large skillet over medium heat.
4. Add the fish fillets and cook each side for 3 to 5 minutes until golden brown and cooked through.
5. Divide the fillets among two plates and spoon half of the prepared salsa onto each fillet. Serve the fish alongside the lime wedges.

Baked Halibut Steaks with Vegetables

Prep time: 15 minutes | Cook time: 20 minutes
Serves 4

2 teaspoon olive oil, divided
1 clove garlic, peeled and minced
½ cup minced onion
1 cup diced zucchini
2 cups diced fresh tomatoes
2 tablespoons chopped fresh

basil
¼ teaspoon salt
¼ teaspoon ground black pepper
4 (6-ounce / 170-g) halibut
steaks
¹/₃ cup crumbled feta cheese

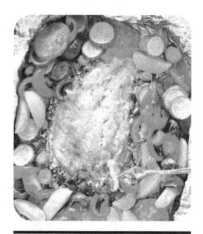

1. Preheat oven to 450ºF (235ºC). Coat a shallow baking dish lightly with 1 teaspoon of olive oil.
2. In a medium saucepan, heat the remaining 1 teaspoon of olive oil.
3. Add the garlic, onion, and zucchini and mix well. Cook for 5 minutes, stirring occasionally, or until the zucchini is softened.
4. Remove the saucepan from the heat and stir in the tomatoes, basil, salt, and pepper.
5. Place the halibut steaks in the coated baking dish in a single layer. Spread the zucchini mixture evenly over the steaks. Scatter the top with feta cheese.
6. Bake in the preheated oven for about 15 minutes, or until the fish flakes when pressed lightly with a fork. Serve hot.

Tip: To make this a complete meal, serve it with roasted potatoes, sautéed asparagus, roasted vegetables, or even a green salad.

Per Serving
calories: 258 | fat: 7.6g
protein: 38.6g | carbs: 6.5g
fiber: 1.2g | sodium: 384mg

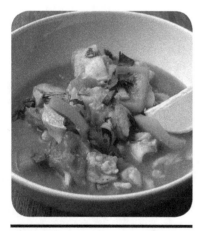

Tip: If you prefer a bit of heat, you could add a bit of chiles.

Per Serving
calories: 276 | fat: 20.9g
protein: 14.2g | carbs: 6.8g
fiber: 3.0g | sodium: 226mg

Spicy Haddock Stew

Prep time: 15 minutes | Cook time: 35 minutes
Serves 6

¼ cup coconut oil
1 tablespoon minced garlic
1 onion, chopped
2 celery stalks, chopped
½ fennel bulb, thinly sliced
1 carrot, diced
1 sweet potato, diced
1 (15-ounce / 425-g) can low-

sodium diced tomatoes
1 cup coconut milk
1 cup low-sodium chicken broth
¼ teaspoon red pepper flakes
12 ounces (340 g) haddock, cut
into 1-inch chunks
2 tablespoons chopped fresh
cilantro, for garnish

1. In a large saucepan, heat the coconut oil over medium-high heat.
2. Add the garlic, onion, and celery and sauté for about 4 minutes, stirring occasionally, or until they are tender.
3. Stir in the fennel bulb, carrot, and sweet potato and sauté for 4 minutes more.
4. Add the diced tomatoes, coconut milk, chicken broth, and red pepper flakes and stir to incorporate, then bring the mixture to a boil.
5. Once it starts to boil, reduce the heat to low, and bring to a simmer for about 15 minutes, or until the vegetables are fork-tender.
6. Add the haddock chunks and continue simmering for about 10 minutes, or until the fish is cooked through.
7. Sprinkle the cilantro on top for garnish before serving.

Cioppino (Seafood Tomato Stew)

Prep time: 10 minutes | Cook time: 20 minutes
Serves 2

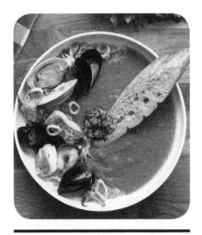

2 tablespoons olive oil
½ small onion, diced
½ green pepper, diced
2 teaspoons dried basil
2 teaspoons dried oregano
½ cup dry white wine
1 (14.5-ounce / 411-g) can diced tomatoes with basil
1 (8-ounce / 227-g) can no-salt-added tomato sauce

1 (6.5-ounce / 184-g) can minced clams with their juice
8 ounces (227 g) peeled, deveined raw shrimp
4 ounces (113 g) any white fish (a thick piece works best)
3 tablespoons fresh parsley
Salt and freshly ground black pepper, to taste

1. In a Dutch oven, heat the olive oil over medium heat.
2. Sauté the onion and green pepper for 5 minutes, or until tender.
3. Stir in the basil, oregano, wine, diced tomatoes, and tomato sauce and bring to a boil.
4. Once boiling, reduce the heat to low and bring to a simmer for 5 minutes.
5. Add the clams, shrimp, and fish and cook for about 10 minutes, or until the shrimp are pink and cooked through.
6. Scatter with the parsley and add the salt and black pepper to taste.
7. Remove from the heat and serve warm.

Tip: You can prepare the base of this stew in advance, but do not stir in the fish until just before serving.

Per Serving
calories: 221 | fat: 7.7g
protein: 23.1g | carbs: 10.9g
fiber: 4.2g | sodium: 720mg

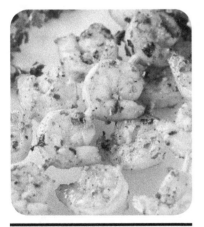

Lemon Grilled Shrimp

Prep time: 20 minutes | Cook time: 4 to 6 minutes
Serves 4

2 tablespoons garlic, minced
3 tablespoons fresh Italian parsley, finely chopped
¼ cup extra-virgin olive oil
½ cup lemon juice
1 teaspoon salt
2 pounds (907 g) jumbo shrimp (21 to 25), peeled and deveined

Special Equipment:
4 skewers, soaked in water for at least 30 minutes

1. Whisk together the garlic, parsley, olive oil, lemon juice, and salt in a large bowl.
2. Add the shrimp to the bowl and toss well, making sure the shrimp are coated in the marinade. Set aside to sit for 15 minutes.
3. When ready, skewer the shrimps by piercing through the center. You can place about 5 to 6 shrimps on each skewer.
4. Preheat the grill to high heat.
5. Grill the shrimp for 4 to 6 minutes, flipping the shrimp halfway through, or until the shrimp are pink on the outside and opaque in the center.
6. Serve hot.

Tip: You can try adding 1 teaspoon paprika to the marinade for added color and flavor. To save time, you can marinate the shrimp ahead of time.

Per Serving
calories: 401 | fat: 17.8g
protein: 56.9g | carbs: 3.9g
fiber: 0g | sodium: 1223mg

Garlic Shrimp with Mushrooms

Prep time: 10 minutes | Cook time: 15 minutes
Serves 4

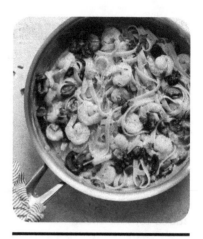

1 pound (454 g) fresh shrimp, peeled, deveined, and patted dry
1 teaspoon salt
1 cup extra-virgin olive oil
8 large garlic cloves, thinly sliced
4 ounces (113 g) sliced mushrooms (shiitake, baby bella, or button)
½ teaspoon red pepper flakes
¼ cup chopped fresh flat-leaf Italian parsley

1. In a bowl, season the shrimp with salt. Set aside.
2. Heat the olive oil in a large skillet over medium-low heat.
3. Add the garlic and cook for 3 to 4 minutes until fragrant, stirring occasionally.
4. Sauté the mushrooms for 5 minutes, or until they start to exude their juices.
5. Stir in the shrimp and sprinkle with red pepper flakes and sauté for 3 to 4 minutes more, or until the shrimp start to turn pink.
6. Remove the skillet from the heat and add the parsley. Stir to combine and serve warm.

Tips: If you have any leftovers, you can serve with mixed greens. If you want to make an easy vinaigrette, you can pour 1 to 2 tablespoons lemon juice or red wine vinegar into the garlic oil.

Per Serving
calories: 619 | fat: 55.5g
protein: 24.1g | carbs: 3.7g
fiber: 0g | sodium: 735mg

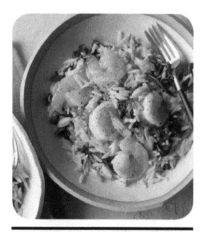

Lemony Shrimp with Orzo Salad

Prep time: 10 minutes | Cook time: 22 minutes
Serves 4

1 cup orzo
1 hothouse cucumber, deseeded and chopped
½ cup finely diced red onion
2 tablespoons extra-virgin olive oil
2 pounds (907 g) shrimp, peeled and deveined
3 lemons, juiced
Salt and freshly ground black pepper, to taste
¾ cup crumbled feta cheese
2 tablespoons dried dill
1 cup chopped fresh flat-leaf parsley

Tips: To add more flavors to this meal, try adding halved cherry tomatoes to the salad. And you can serve the shrimp with grilled vegetables or over a bed of lettuce.

Per Serving
calories: 565 | fat: 17.8g
protein: 63.3g | carbs: 43.9g
fiber: 4.1g | sodium: 2225mg

1. Bring a large pot of water to a boil. Add the orzo and cook covered for 15 to 18 minutes, or until the orzo is tender. Transfer to a colander to drain and set aside to cool.
2. Mix the cucumber and red onion in a bowl. Set aside.
3. Heat the olive oil in a medium skillet over medium heat until it shimmers.
4. Reduce the heat, add the shrimp, and cook each side for 2 minutes until cooked through.
5. Add the cooked shrimp to the bowl of cucumber and red onion. Mix in the cooked orzo and lemon juice and toss to combine. Sprinkle with salt and pepper. Scatter the top with the feta cheese and dill. Garnish with the parsley and serve immediately.

Avocado Shrimp Ceviche

Prep time: 15 minutes | Cook time: 0 minutes
Serves 4

1 pound (454 g) fresh shrimp, peeled, deveined, and cut in half lengthwise
1 small red or yellow bell pepper, cut into ½-inch chunks
½ small red onion, cut into thin slivers
½ English cucumber, peeled and cut into ½-inch chunks
¼ cup chopped fresh cilantro
½ cup extra-virgin olive oil
¹/₃ cup freshly squeezed lime juice
2 tablespoons freshly squeezed clementine juice
2 tablespoons freshly squeezed lemon juice
1 teaspoon salt
½ teaspoon freshly ground black pepper
2 ripe avocados, peeled, pitted, and cut into ½-inch chunks

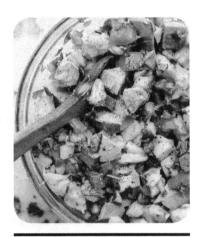

1. Place the shrimp, bell pepper, red onion, cucumber, and cilantro in a large bowl and toss to combine.
2. In a separate bowl, stir together the olive oil, lime, clementine, and lemon juice, salt, and black pepper until smooth. Pour the mixture into the bowl of shrimp and vegetable mixture and toss until they are completely coated.
3. Cover the bowl with plastic wrap and transfer to the refrigerator to marinate for at least 2 hours, or up to 8 hours.
4. When ready, stir in the avocado chunks and toss to incorporate. Serve immediately.

Tip: If the clementine juice isn't available, the orange juice will work, too. And you can add the parsley to the marinade for added flavor.

Per Serving
calories: 496 | fat: 39.5g
protein: 25.3g | carbs: 13.8g
fiber: 6.0g | sodium: 755mg

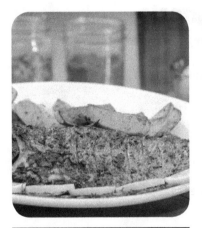

Tip: To make this a complete meal, serve the grilled sea bass with rice and grilled or steamed vegetables.

Per Serving
calories: 200 | fat: 10.3g
protein: 26.9g | carbs: 0.6g
fiber: 0.1g | sodium: 105mg

Mediterranean Grilled Sea Bass

Prep time: 20 minutes | Cook time: 20 minutes
Serves 6

¼ teaspoon onion powder
¼ teaspoon garlic powder
¼ teaspoon paprika
Lemon pepper and sea salt to taste
2 pounds (907 g) sea bass
3 tablespoons extra-virgin olive oil, divided
2 large cloves garlic, chopped
1 tablespoon chopped Italian flat leaf parsley

1. Preheat the grill to high heat.
2. Place the onion powder, garlic powder, paprika, lemon pepper, and sea salt in a large bowl and stir to combine.
3. Dredge the fish in the spice mixture, turning until well coated.
4. Heat 2 tablespoon of olive oil in a small skillet. Add the garlic and parsley and cook for 1 to 2 minutes, stirring occasionally. Remove the skillet from the heat and set aside.
5. Brush the grill grates lightly with remaining 1 tablespoon olive oil.
6. Grill the fish for about 7 minutes. Flip the fish and drizzle with the garlic mixture and cook for an additional 7 minutes, or until the fish flakes when pressed lightly with a fork.
7. Serve hot.

Orange Flavored Scallops

Prep time: 10 minutes | Cook time: 10 minutes
Serves 4

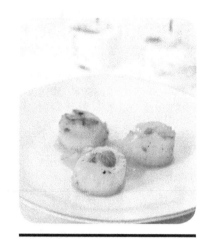

2 pounds (907 g) sea scallops, patted dry
Sea salt and freshly ground black pepper, to taste
2 tablespoons extra-virgin olive oil
1 tablespoon minced garlic
¼ cup freshly squeezed orange juice
1 teaspoon orange zest
2 teaspoons chopped fresh thyme, for garnish

1. In a bowl, lightly season the scallops with salt and pepper. Set aside.
2. Heat the olive oil in a large skillet over medium-high heat until it shimmers.
3. Add the garlic and sauté for about 3 minutes, or until fragrant.
4. Stir in the seasoned scallops and sear each side for about 4 minutes, or until the scallops are browned.
5. Remove the scallops from the heat to a plate and set aside.
6. Add the orange juice and zest to the skillet, scraping up brown bits from bottom of skillet.
7. Drizzle the sauce over the scallops and garnish with the thyme before serving.

Tip: To make this a complete meal, you can serve it with cooked rice or quinoa.

Per Serving
calories: 266 | fat: 7.6g
protein: 38.1g | carbs: 7.9g
fiber: 0g | sodium: 360mg

Chapter 10 Fruits and Desserts

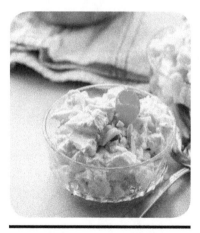

Apple and Berries Ambrosia

Prep time: 15 minutes | Cook time: 0 minutes
Serves 4

2 cups unsweetened coconut milk, chilled
2 tablespoons raw honey
1 apple, peeled, cored, and chopped
2 cups fresh raspberries
2 cups fresh blueberries

1. Spoon the chilled milk in a large bowl, then mix in the honey. Stir to mix well.
2. Then mix in the remaining ingredients. Stir to coat the fruits well and serve immediately.

Tip: You can also try this recipe out with any kinds of fruit chunks, such as pears, peaches, bananas, nectarines, or melons.

Per Serving
calories: 386 | fat: 21.1g
protein: 4.2g | carbs: 45.9g
fiber: 11.0g | sodium: 16mg

Banana, Cranberry, and Oat Bars

Prep time: 15 minutes | Cook time: 40 minutes
Makes 16 bars

2 tablespoon extra-virgin olive oil
2 medium ripe bananas, mashed
½ cup almond butter
½ cup maple syrup
1/3 cup dried cranberries
1½ cups old-fashioned rolled oats

¼ cup oat flour
¼ cup ground flaxseed
¼ teaspoon ground cloves
½ cup shredded coconut
½ teaspoon ground cinnamon
1 teaspoon vanilla extract

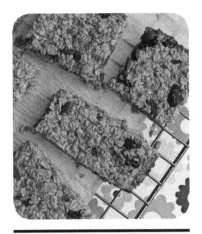

1. Preheat the oven to 400ºF (205ºC). Line a 8-inch square pan with parchment paper, then grease with olive oil.
2. Combine the mashed bananas, almond butter, and maple syrup in a bowl. Stir to mix well.
3. Mix in the remaining ingredients and stir to mix well until thick and sticky.
4. Spread the mixture evenly on the square pan with a spatula, then bake in the preheated oven for 40 minutes or until a toothpick inserted in the center comes out clean.
5. Remove them from the oven and slice into 16 bars to serve.

Tip: Instead of oat flour, you can also use almond flour or coconut flour.

Per Serving
calories: 145 | fat: 7.2g
protein: 3.1g | carbs: 18.9g
fiber: 2.0g | sodium: 3mg

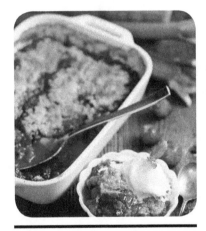

Tip: For more variation, you can replace the berries and rhubarb with plums, pears, or pumpkin, cherry, and sweet potato.

Per Serving
calories: 305 | fat: 22.1g
protein: 3.2g | carbs: 29.8g
fiber: 4.0g | sodium: 3mg

Berry and Rhubarb Cobbler

Prep time: 15 minutes | Cook time: 35 minutes
Serves 8

Cobbler:
1 cup fresh raspberries
2 cups fresh blueberries
1 cup sliced (½-inch) rhubarb pieces

1 tablespoon arrowroot powder
¼ cup unsweetened apple juice
2 tablespoons melted coconut oil
¼ cup raw honey

Topping:
1 cup almond flour
1 tablespoon arrowroot powder
½ cup shredded coconut

¼ cup raw honey
½ cup coconut oil

Make the Cobbler
1. Preheat the oven to 350ºF (180ºC). Grease a baking dish with melted coconut oil.
2. Combine the ingredients for the cobbler in a large bowl. Stir to mix well.
3. Spread the mixture in the single layer on the baking dish. Set aside.

Make the Topping
1. Combine the almond flour, arrowroot powder, and coconut in a bowl. Stir to mix well.
2. Fold in the honey and coconut oil. Stir with a fork until the mixture crumbled.
3. Spread the topping over the cobbler, then bake in the preheated oven for 35 minutes or until frothy and golden brown.
4. Serve immediately.

Citrus Cranberry and Quinoa Energy Bites

Prep time: 25 minutes | Cook time: 0 minutes
Makes 12 bites

30m or less

2 tablespoons almond butter
2 tablespoons maple syrup
¾ cup cooked quinoa
1 tablespoon dried cranberries
1 tablespoon chia seeds

¼ cup ground almonds
¼ cup sesame seeds, toasted
Zest of 1 orange
½ teaspoon vanilla extract

1. Line a baking sheet with parchment paper.
2. Combine the butter and maple syrup in a bowl. Stir to mix well.
3. Fold in the remaining ingredients and stir until the mixture holds together and smooth.
4. Divide the mixture into 12 equal parts, then shape each part into a ball.
5. Arrange the balls on the baking sheet, then refrigerate for at least 15 minutes.
6. Serve chilled.

Tip: How to cook quinoa: Pour the quinoa in a pot, then pour in enough water to cover. Sprinkle with a dash of salt, if needed. Bring to a boil. Reduce the heat to low and simmer for 15 minutes or until the quinoa is tender and the liquid is almost absorbed. Fluffy with a fork and allow to cool before using.

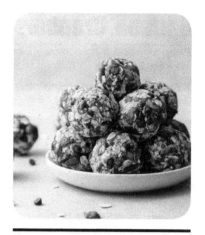

Per Serving (1 bite)
calories: 110 | fat: 10.8g
protein: 3.1g | carbs: 4.9g
fiber: 3.0g | sodium: 211mg

Chocolate, Almond, and Cherry Clusters

Prep time: 15 minutes | Cook time: 3 minutes
Makes 10 clusters

30m or less   5-ingre

1 cup dark chocolate (60% cocoa or higher), chopped
1 tablespoon coconut oil
½ cup dried cherries
1 cup roasted salted almonds

1. Line a baking sheet with parchment paper.
2. Melt the chocolate and coconut oil in a saucepan for 3 minutes. Stir constantly.
3. Turn off the heat and mix in the cherries and almonds.
4. Drop the mixture on the baking sheet with a spoon. Place the sheet in the refrigerator and chill for at least 1 hour or until firm.
5. Serve chilled.

Tip: You can also melt the chocolate and coconut oil in the microwave for 1 minute.

Per Serving
calories: 197 | fat: 13.2g
protein: 4.1g | carbs: 17.8g
fiber: 4.0g | sodium: 57mg

Chocolate and Avocado Mousse

Prep time: 40 minutes | Cook time: 5 minutes
Serves 4 to 6

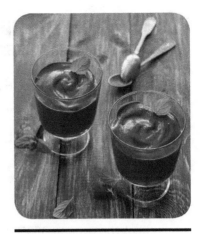

8 ounces (227 g) dark chocolate (60% cocoa or higher), chopped
¼ cup unsweetened coconut milk
2 tablespoons coconut oil
2 ripe avocados, deseeded
¼ cup raw honey
Sea salt, to taste

1. Put the chocolate in a saucepan. Pour in the coconut milk and add the coconut oil.
2. Cook for 3 minutes or until the chocolate and coconut oil melt. Stir constantly.
3. Put the avocado in a food processor, then drizzle with honey and melted chocolate. Pulse to combine until smooth.
4. Pour the mixture in a serving bowl, then sprinkle with salt. Refrigerate to chill for 30 minutes and serve.

Tip: You can chopped the avocado in chunks or slices before pulsing in the food processor to make the purée process easier.

Per Serving
calories: 654 | fat: 46.8g
protein: 7.2g | carbs: 55.9g
fiber: 9.0g | sodium: 112mg

Coconut Blueberries with Brown Rice

Prep time: 55 minutes | Cook time: 10 minutes
Serves 4

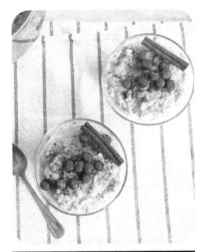

1 cup fresh blueberries
2 cups unsweetened coconut milk
1 teaspoon ground ginger
¼ cup maple syrup
Sea salt, to taste
2 cups cooked brown rice

1. Put all the ingredients, except for the brown rice, in a pot. Stir to combine well.
2. Cook over medium-high heat for 7 minutes or until the blueberries are tender.
3. Pour in the brown rice and cook for 3 more minute or until the rice is soft. Stir constantly.
4. Serve immediately.

Tip: How to cook the brown rice: Pour the rinsed brown rice in a pot, then pour in enough water to cover the rice about 1-inch. Sprinkle with salt, if desired. Bring to a boil. Reduce the heat to low and simmer for 45 minutes or until the rice is tender. Drain the cooked rice and fluff with a fork. Allow to cool before using.

Per Serving
calories: 470 | fat: 24.8g
protein: 6.2g | carbs: 60.1g
fiber: 5.0g | sodium: 75mg

Easy Blueberry and Oat Crisp

Prep time: 15 minutes | Cook time: 20 minutes
Serves 4

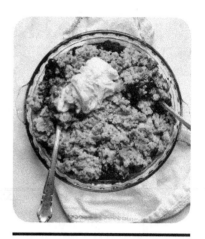

2 tablespoons coconut oil, melted, plus additional for greasing
4 cups fresh blueberries
Juice of ½ lemon
2 teaspoons lemon zest
¼ cup maple syrup
1 cup gluten-free rolled oats
½ cup chopped pecans
½ teaspoon ground cinnamon
Sea salt, to taste

1. Preheat the oven to 350ºF (180ºC). Grease a baking sheet with coconut oil.
2. Combine the blueberries, lemon juice and zest, and maple syrup in a bowl. Stir to mix well, then spread the mixture on the baking sheet.
3. Combine the remaining ingredients in a small bowl. Stir to mix well. Pour the mixture over the blueberries mixture.
4. Bake in the preheated oven for 20 minutes or until the oats are golden brown.
5. Serve immediately with spoons.

Tip: You can use quinoa to replace the rolled oats, if needed.

Per Serving
calories: 496 | fat: 32.9g
protein: 5.1g | carbs: 50.8g
fiber: 7.0g | sodium: 41mg

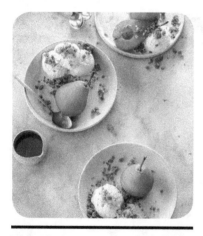

Glazed Pears with Hazelnuts

Prep time: 10 minutes | Cook time: 20 minutes
Serves 4

4 pears, peeled, cored, and quartered lengthwise
1 cup apple juice
1 tablespoon grated fresh ginger
½ cup pure maple syrup
¼ cup chopped hazelnuts

1. Put the pears in a pot, then pour in the apple juice. Bring to a boil over medium-high heat, then reduce the heat to medium-low. Stir constantly.
2. Cover and simmer for an additional 15 minutes or until the pears are tender.
3. Meanwhile, combine the ginger and maple syrup in a saucepan. Bring to a boil over medium-high heat. Stir frequently. Turn off the heat and transfer the syrup to a small bowl and let sit until ready to use.
4. Transfer the pears in a large serving bowl with a slotted spoon, then top the pears with syrup.
5. Spread the hazelnuts over the pears and serve immediately.

Tip: If you want to add a milky flavor for the pears, you can pour in 1 cup of unsweetened almond milk in the pot and boil with peas and apple juice.

Per Serving
calories: 287 | fat: 3.1g
protein: 2.2g | carbs: 66.9g
fiber: 7.0g | sodium: 8mg

Lemony Blackberry Granita

Prep time: 10 minutes | Cook time: 0 minutes
Serves 4

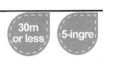
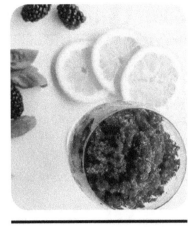

1 pound (454 g) fresh blackberries
1 teaspoon chopped fresh thyme
¼ cup freshly squeezed lemon juice
½ cup raw honey
½ cup water

1. Put all the ingredients in a food processor, then pulse to purée.
2. Pour the mixture through a sieve into a baking dish. Discard the seeds remain in the sieve.
3. Put the baking dish in the freezer for 2 hours. Remove the dish from the refrigerator and stir to break any frozen parts.
4. Return the dish back to the freezer for an hour, then stir to break any frozen parts again.
5. Return the dish to the freezer for 4 hours until the granita is completely frozen.
6. Remove it from the freezer and mash to serve.

Tip: You can mix other kinds of the berries, such as blueberries or strawberries, with blackberries for a magic mixed flavor.

Per Serving
calories: 183 | fat: 1.1g
protein: 2.2g | carbs: 45.9g
fiber: 6.0g | sodium: 6mg

Lemony Tea and Chia Pudding

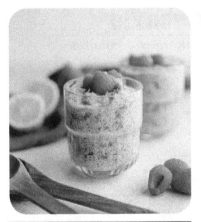

Prep time: 30 minutes | Cook time: 0 minutes
Serves 3 to 4

2 teaspoons matcha green tea powder (optional)
2 tablespoons ground chia seeds
1 to 2 dates
2 cups unsweetened coconut milk
Zest and juice of 1 lime

1. Put all the ingredients in a food processor and pulse until creamy and smooth.
2. Pour the mixture in a bowl, then wrap in plastic. Store in the refrigerator for at least 20 minutes, then serve chilled.

Tip: Dates are used as sugar, so you can replace them with 1 tablespoon of coconut sugar / maple syrup, or 15 drops liquid stevia.

Per Serving
calories: 225 | fat: 20.1g
protein: 3.2g | carbs: 5.9g
fiber: 5.0g | sodium: 314mg

Sweet Spiced Pumpkin Pudding

Prep time: 2 hours 10 minutes | Cook time: 0 minutes
Serves 6

1 cup pure pumpkin purée
2 cups unsweetened coconut milk
1 teaspoon ground cinnamon
¼ teaspoon ground nutmeg
½ teaspoon ground ginger
Pinch cloves
¼ cup pure maple syrup
2 tablespoons chopped pecans, for garnish

1. Combine all the ingredients, except for the chopped pecans, in a large bowl. Stir to mix well.
2. Wrap the bowl in plastic and refrigerate for at least 2 hours.
3. Remove the bowl from the refrigerator and discard the plastic. Spread the pudding with pecans and serve chilled.

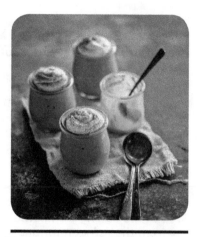

Tip: Instead of pumpkin purée, you can use the same amount of puréed butternut squash or sweet potato to replace it.

Per Serving
calories: 249 | fat: 21.1g
protein: 2.8g | carbs: 17.2g
fiber: 3.0g | sodium: 46mg

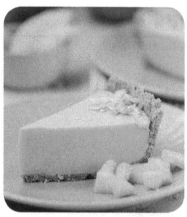

Tip: If you have mango allergy, then you can replace the mangoes with peach chunks or sliced apples.

Per Serving (1 slice)
calories: 426 | fat: 28.2g
protein: 8.1g | carbs: 14.9g
fiber: 6.0g | sodium: 174mg

Mango and Coconut Frozen Pie

Prep time: 1 hour 10 minutes | Cook time: 0 minutes
Serves 8

Crust:
1 cup cashews
½ cup rolled oats
1 cup soft pitted dates

Filling:
2 large mangoes, peeled and chopped
½ cup unsweetened shredded coconut
1 cup unsweetened coconut milk
½ cup water

1. Combine the ingredients for the crust in a food processor. Pulse to combine well.
2. Pour the mixture in an 8-inch springform pan, then press to coat the bottom. Set aside.
3. Combine the ingredients for the filling in the food processor, then pulse to purée until smooth.
4. Pour the filling over the crust, then use a spatula to spread the filling evenly. Put the pan in the freeze for 30 minutes.
5. Remove the pan from the freezer and allow to sit for 15 minutes under room temperature before serving.

Mini Nuts and Fruits Crumble

Prep time: 15 minutes | Cook time: 15 minutes
Serves 6

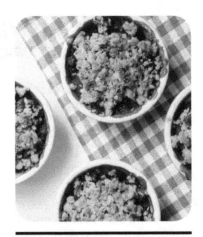

Topping:
¼ cup coarsely chopped hazelnuts
1 cup coarsely chopped walnuts
1 teaspoon ground cinnamon
Sea salt, to taste
1 tablespoon melted coconut oil

Filling:
6 fresh figs, quartered
2 nectarines, pitted and sliced
1 cup fresh blueberries
2 teaspoons lemon zest
½ cup raw honey
1 teaspoon vanilla extract

Make the Topping:
1. Combine the ingredients for the topping in a bowl. Stir to mix well. Set aside until ready to use.

Make the Filling:
1. Preheat the oven to 375ºF (190ºC).
2. Combine the ingredients for the fillings in a bowl. Stir to mix well.
3. Divide the filling in six ramekins, then divide and top with nut topping.
4. Bake in the preheated oven for 15 minutes or until the topping is lightly browned and the filling is frothy.
5. Serve immediately.

Tip: You can use coconut sugar, pure date sugar, maple sugar, or liquid stevia to replace the raw honey, if needed.

Per Serving
calories: 336 | fat: 18.8g
protein: 6.3g | carbs: 41.9g
fiber: 6.0g | sodium: 31mg

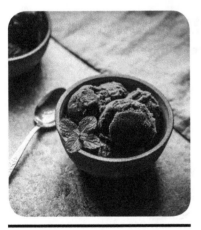

Mint Banana Chocolate Sorbet

Prep time: 4 hours 5 minutes | Cook time: 0 minutes
Serves 1

1 frozen banana
1 tablespoon almond butter
2 tablespoons minced fresh mint
2 to 3 tablespoons dark chocolate chips (60% cocoa or higher)
2 to 3 tablespoons goji (optional)

1. Put the banana, butter, and mint in a food processor. Pulse to purée until creamy and smooth.
2. Add the chocolate and goji, then pulse for several more times to combine well.
3. Pour the mixture in a bowl or a ramekin, then freeze for at least 4 hours before serving chilled.

Tip: You can pour ¼ cup of almond milk when purée the banana, butter, and mint to help them to purée.

Per Serving
calories: 213 | fat: 9.8g
protein: 3.1g | carbs: 2.9g
fiber: 4.0g | sodium: 155mg

Pecan and Carrot Cake

Prep time: 15 minutes | Cook time: 45 minutes
Serves 12

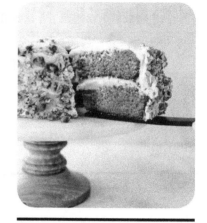

½ cup coconut oil, at room
temperature, plus more for
greasing the baking dish
2 teaspoons pure vanilla extract
¼ cup pure maple syrup
6 eggs
½ cup coconut flour

1 teaspoon baking powder
1 teaspoon baking soda
½ teaspoon ground nutmeg
1 teaspoon ground cinnamon
⅛ teaspoon sea salt
½ cup chopped pecans
3 cups finely grated carrots

1. Preheat the oven to 350ºF (180ºC). Grease a 13-by-9-inch
   baking dish with coconut oil.
2. Combine the vanilla extract, maple syrup, and ½ cup of coconut
   oil in a large bowl. Stir to mix well.
3. Break the eggs in the bowl and whisk to combine well. Set aside.
4. Combine the coconut flour, baking powder, baking soda, nutmeg,
   cinnamon, and salt in a separate bowl. Stir to mix well.
5. Make a well in the center of the flour mixture, then pour the egg
   mixture into the well. Stir to combine well.
6. Add the pecans and carrots to the bowl and toss to mix well.
   Pour the mixture in the single layer on the baking dish.
7. Bake in the preheated oven for 45 minutes or until puffed and
   the cake spring back when lightly press with your fingers.
8. Remove the cake from the oven. Allow to cool for at least 15
   minutes, then serve.

Tip: If you have nut allergies,
just omit the pecans, or you
can replace it with goji or
cherries.

Per Serving
calories: 255 | fat: 21.2g
protein: 5.1g | carbs: 12.8g
fiber: 2.0g | sodium: 202mg

Raspberry Yogurt Basted Cantaloupe

Prep time: 15 minutes | Cook time: 0 minutes
Serves 6

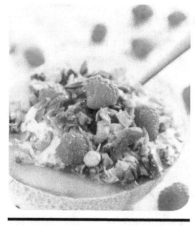

2 cups fresh raspberries, mashed
1 cup plain coconut yogurt
½ teaspoon vanilla extract
1 cantaloupe, peeled and sliced
½ cup toasted coconut flakes

1. Combine the mashed raspberries with yogurt and vanilla extract
   in a small bowl. Stir to mix well.
2. Place the cantaloupe slices on a platter, then top with raspberry
   mixture and spread with toasted coconut.
3. Serve immediately.

Tip: How to toast the coconut:
Preheat the oven to 325ºF
(163ºC), then put the coconut
flakes on a baking sheet
directly. Bake in the preheated
oven for 5 minutes or until
lightly browned.

Per Serving
calories: 75 | fat: 4.1g
protein: 1.2g | carbs: 10.9g
fiber: 6.0g | sodium: 36mg

Simple Apple Compote

Prep time: 15 minutes | Cook time: 10 minutes
Serves 4

6 apples, peeled, cored, and chopped
¼ cup raw honey
1 teaspoon ground cinnamon
¼ cup apple juice
Sea salt, to taste

1. Put all the ingredients in a stockpot. Stir to mix well, then cook over medium-high heat for 10 minutes or until the apples are glazed by honey and lightly saucy. Stir constantly.
2. Serve immediately.

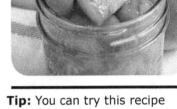

Tip: You can try this recipe with different fruits, such as pears or peaches.

Per Serving
calories: 246 | fat: 0.9g
protein: 1.2g | carbs: 66.3g
fiber: 9.0g | sodium: 62mg

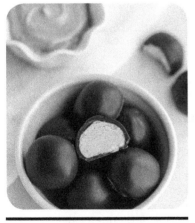

Tip: For more flavor, you can glaze the chilled balls with melted dark chocolate (60% cocoa or higher) and sprinkle with mashed nuts.

Per Serving (1 ball)
calories: 146 | fat: 8.1g
protein: 4.2g | carbs: 16.9g
fiber: 1.0g | sodium: 70mg

Simple Peanut Butter and Chocolate Balls

Prep time: 45 minutes | Cook time: 0 minutes
Serves 15 balls

¾ cup creamy peanut butter
¼ cup unsweetened cocoa powder
2 tablespoons softened almond butter
½ teaspoon vanilla extract
1¾ cups maple sugar

1. Line a baking sheet with parchment paper.
2. Combine all the ingredients in a bowl. Stir to mix well.
3. Divide the mixture into 15 parts and shape each part into a 1-inch ball.
4. Arrange the balls on the baking sheet and refrigerate for at least 30 minutes, then serve chilled.

Simple Spiced Sweet Pecans

Prep time: 4 minutes | Cook time: 17 minutes
Serves 4

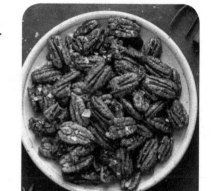

1 cup pecan halves
3 tablespoons almond butter
1 teaspoon ground cinnamon
½ teaspoon ground nutmeg
¼ cup raw honey
¼ teaspoon sea salt

1. Preheat the oven to 350ºF (180ºC). Line a baking sheet with parchment paper.
2. Combine all the ingredients in a bowl. Stir to mix well, then spread the mixture in the single layer on the baking sheet with a spatula.
3. Bake in the preheated oven for 16 minutes or until the pecan halves are well browned.
4. Serve immediately.

Tip: Instead of almond butter, you can also use peanut butter.

Per Serving
calories: 324 | fat: 29.8g
protein: 3.2g | carbs: 13.9g
fiber: 4.0g | sodium: 180mg

Chapter 11 Sauces, Dips, and Dressings

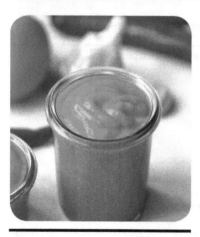

Hot Pepper Sauce

Prep time: 10 minutes | Cook time: 20 minutes
Makes 4 cups

2 red hot fresh chiles, deseeded
2 dried chiles
2 garlic cloves, peeled
½ small yellow onion, roughly chopped
2 cups water
2 cups white vinegar

1. Place all the ingredients except the vinegar in a medium saucepan over medium heat. Allow to simmer for 20 minutes until softened.
2. Transfer the mixture to a food processor or blender. Stir in the vinegar and pulse until very smooth.
3. Serve immediately or transfer to a sealed container and refrigerate for up to 3 months.

Tip: If you prefer a milder hot sauce, you can use a seeded jalapeño pepper or serrano pepper instead of the red chiles.

Per Serving (2 tablespoons)
calories: 20 | fat: 1.2g
protein: 0.6g | carbs: 4.4g
fiber: 0.6g | sodium: 12mg

Lemon-Tahini Sauce

Prep time: 10 minutes | Cook time: 0 minutes
Makes 1 cup

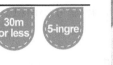

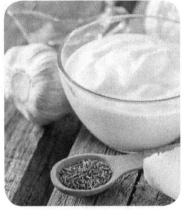

½ cup tahini
1 garlic clove, minced
Juice and zest of 1 lemon
½ teaspoon salt, plus more as needed
½ cup warm water, plus more as needed

1. Combine the tahini and garlic in a small bowl.
2. Add the lemon juice and zest and salt to the bowl and stir to mix well.
3. Fold in the warm water and whisk until well combined and creamy. Feel free to add more warm water if you like a thinner consistency.
4. Taste and add additional salt as needed.
5. Store the sauce in a sealed container in the refrigerator for up to 5 days.

Tip: You can make this sauce ahead of time and keep it in the refrigerator. Remember to add a few tablespoons of hot water and stir well before using.

Per Serving (¼ cup)
calories: 179 | fat: 15.5g
protein: 5.1g | carbs: 6.8g
fiber: 3.0g | sodium: 324mg

Peri-Peri Sauce

Prep time: 10 minutes | Cook time: 5 minutes
Serves 4

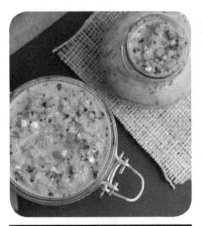

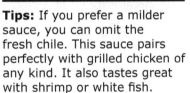

1 tomato, chopped
1 red onion, chopped
1 red bell pepper, deseeded and chopped
1 red chile, deseeded and chopped
4 garlic cloves, minced
2 tablespoons extra-virgin olive oil
Juice of 1 lemon
1 tablespoon dried oregano
1 tablespoon smoked paprika
1 teaspoon sea salt

1. Process all the ingredients in a food processor or a blender until smooth.
2. Transfer the mixture to a small saucepan over medium-high heat and bring to a boil, stirring often.
3. Reduce the heat to medium and allow to simmer for 5 minutes until heated through.
4. You can store the sauce in an airtight container in the refrigerator for up to 5 days.

Tips: If you prefer a milder sauce, you can omit the fresh chile. This sauce pairs perfectly with grilled chicken of any kind. It also tastes great with shrimp or white fish.

Per Serving
calories: 98 | fat: 6.5g
protein: 1.0g | carbs: 7.8g
fiber: 3.0g | sodium: 295mg

Peanut Sauce with Honey

Prep time: 5 minutes | Cook time: 0 minutes
Serves 4

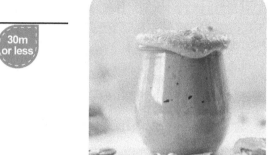

¼ cup peanut butter
1 tablespoon peeled and grated fresh ginger
1 tablespoon honey
1 tablespoon low-sodium soy sauce
1 garlic clove, minced
Juice of 1 lime
Pinch red pepper flakes

1. Whisk together all the ingredients in a small bowl until well incorporated.
2. Transfer to an airtight container and refrigerate for up to 5 days.

Tip: The peanut butter can be substituted with the cashew butter or almond butter. This sauce works great with stir-fries, and it also can be used as a dip for the chicken fingers or topping for beef or seafood.

Per Serving
calories: 117 | fat: 7.6g
protein: 4.1g | carbs: 8.8g
fiber: 1.0g | sodium: 136mg

Cilantro-Tomato Salsa

Prep time: 10 minutes | Cook time: 0 minutes
Serves 6

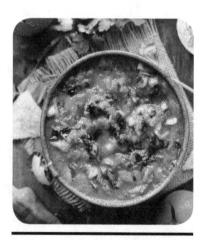

2 or 3 medium, ripe tomatoes, diced
1 serrano pepper, seeded and minced
½ red onion, minced
¼ cup minced fresh cilantro
Juice of 1 lime
¼ teaspoon salt, plus more as needed

1. Place the tomatoes, serrano pepper, onion, cilantro, lime juice, and salt in a small bowl and mix well.
2. Taste and add additional salt, if needed.
3. Store in an airtight container in the refrigerator for up to 3 days.

Tip: This salsa can be used as a dip with chips, a topping on tacos or baked potatoes, or a sauce for grilled fish and meats.

Per Serving (¼ cup)
calories: 17 | fat: 0g protein: 1.0g | carbs: 3.9g fiber: 1.0g | sodium: 83mg

Cheesy Pea Pesto

Prep time: 5 minutes | Cook time: 0 minutes
Serves 4

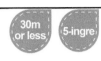

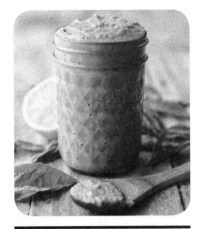

½ cup fresh green peas
½ cup grated Parmesan cheese
¼ cup extra-virgin olive oil
¼ cup pine nuts
¼ cup fresh basil leaves
2 garlic cloves, minced
¼ teaspoon sea salt

1. Add all the ingredients to a food processor or blender and pulse until the nuts are chopped finely.
2. Transfer to an airtight container and refrigerate for up to 2 days. You can also store it in ice cube trays in the freezer for up to 6 months.

Per Serving
calories: 247 | fat: 22.8g
protein: 7.1g | carbs: 4.8g
fiber: 1.0g | sodium: 337mg

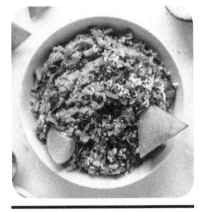

Tips: If you prefer a chunkier guacamole, leave some larger pieces of avocados when you are mashing it. If you prefer a smooth guacamole, you can purée the avocados in a blender. This guacamole can be used as a dip for veggies and a spread on sandwiches.

Per Serving (¼ cup)
calories: 81 | fat: 6.8g
protein: 1.1g | carbs: 5.7g
fiber: 3.0g | sodium: 83mg

Guacamole

Prep time: 10 minutes | Cook time: 0 minutes
Serves 6

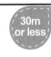

2 large avocados
¼ white onion, finely diced
1 small, firm tomato, finely diced
¼ cup finely chopped fresh cilantro
2 tablespoons freshly squeezed lime juice
¼ teaspoon salt
Freshly ground black pepper, to taste

1. Slice the avocados in half and remove the pits. Using a large spoon to scoop out the flesh and add to a medium bowl.
2. Mash the avocado flesh with the back of a fork, or until a uniform consistency is achieved. Add the onion, tomato, cilantro, lime juice, salt, and pepper to the bowl and stir to combine.
3. Serve immediately, or transfer to an airtight container and refrigerate until chilled.

Lentil-Tahini Dip

Prep time: 10 minutes | Cook time: 15 minutes
Makes 3 cups

30m or less | 5-ingre

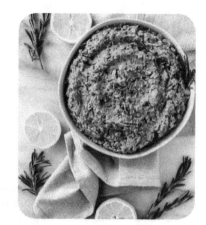

1 cup dried green or brown lentils, rinsed
2½ cups water, divided
1/3 cup tahini
1 garlic clove
½ teaspoon salt, plus more as needed

1. Add the lentils and 2 cups of water to a medium saucepan and bring to a boil over high heat.
2. Once it starts to boil, reduce the heat to low, and then cook for 14 minutes, stirring occasionally, or the lentils become tender but still hold their shape. You can drain any excess liquid.
3. Transfer the lentils to a food processor, along with the remaining water, tahini, garlic, and salt and process until smooth and creamy.
4. Taste and adjust the seasoning if needed. Serve immediately.

Tip: To add more flavors to this dip, garnish it with finely chopped parsley, basil, dill, or rosemary.

Per Serving (¼ cup)
calories: 100 | fat: 3.9g
protein: 5.1g | carbs: 10.7g
fiber: 6.0g | sodium: 106mg

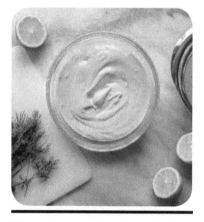

Lemon-Dill Cashew Dip

Prep time: 10 minutes | Cook time: 0 minutes
Makes 1 cup

 30m or less | 5-ingre

¾ cup cashews, soaked in water for at least 4 hours and drained well
¼ cup water
Juice and zest of 1 lemon
2 tablespoons chopped fresh dill
¼ teaspoon salt, plus more as needed

1. Put the cashews, water, lemon juice and zest in a blender and blend until smooth.
2. Add the dill and salt to the blender and blend again.
3. Taste and adjust the seasoning, if needed.
4. Transfer to an airtight container and refrigerate for at least 1 hour to blend the flavors.
5. Serve chilled.

Tips: If you want to make it a nut-free dish, you can substitute the soaked sunflower seeds for the cashews. This dip pairs perfectly with the chili or tacos. It also can be served as a sauce for steamed vegetables or gluten-free toast.

Per Serving (1 tablespoon)
calories: 37 | fat: 2.9g
protein: 1.1g | carbs: 1.9g
fiber: 0g | sodium: 36mg

Creamy Cucumber Dip

Prep time: 10 minutes | Cook time: 0 minutes
Serves 6

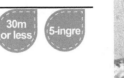

1 medium cucumber, peeled and grated
¼ teaspoon salt
1 cup plain Greek yogurt
2 garlic cloves, minced
1 tablespoon extra-virgin olive oil
1 tablespoon freshly squeezed lemon juice
¼ teaspoon freshly ground black pepper

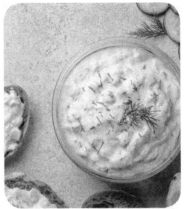

1. Place the grated cucumber in a colander set over a bowl and season with salt. Allow the cucumber to stand for 10 minutes. Using your hands, squeeze out as much liquid from the cucumber as possible. Transfer the grated cucumber to a medium bowl.
2. Add the yogurt, garlic, olive oil, lemon juice, and pepper to the bowl and stir until well blended.
3. Cover the bowl with plastic wrap and refrigerate for at least 2 hours to blend the flavors.
4. Serve chilled.

Tips: For a unique flavor, you can add ½ teaspoon ground cumin to this cucumber dip. This dip perfectly pairs with the veggies, whole-grain pita, and falafel.

Per Serving (¼ cup)
calories: 47 | fat: 2.8g
protein: 4.2g | carbs: 2.7g
fiber: 0g | sodium: 103mg

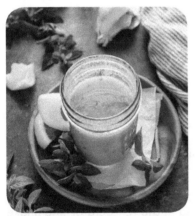

Tips: For a spicy kick, add a pinch of red pepper flakes to this dressing and mix well. If you want to enhance the flavor, you can add some shredded Parmesan cheese.

Per Serving (1 tablespoon)
calories: 80 | fat: 8.6g
protein: 0g | carbs: 0g fiber: 0g | sodium: 51mg

Simple Italian Dressing

Prep time: 5 minutes | Cook time: 0 minutes
Serves 12

½ cup extra-virgin olive oil
¼ cup red wine vinegar
1 teaspoon dried Italian seasoning
1 teaspoon Dijon mustard
¼ teaspoon salt
¼ teaspoon freshly ground black pepper
1 garlic clove, minced

1. Place all the ingredients in a mason jar and cover. Shake vigorously for 1 minute until completely mixed.
2. Store in the refrigerator for up to 1 week.

Ranch-Style Cauliflower Dressing

Prep time: 10 minutes | Cook time: 0 minutes
Serves 8

2 cups frozen cauliflower, thawed
½ cup unsweetened plain almond milk
2 tablespoons apple cider vinegar
2 tablespoons extra-virgin olive oil
1 garlic clove, peeled
2 teaspoons finely chopped fresh parsley
2 teaspoons finely chopped scallions (both white and green parts)
1 teaspoon finely chopped fresh dill
½ teaspoon onion powder
½ teaspoon Dijon mustard
½ teaspoon salt
¼ teaspoon freshly ground black pepper

1. Place all the ingredients in a blender and pulse until creamy and smooth.
2. Serve immediately, or transfer to an airtight container to refrigerate for up to 3 days.

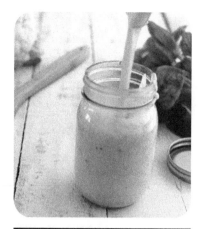

Tips: To add more flavors to this dressing, you can add the thyme, oregano, and shallots. This dressing perfectly goes with the green salads and grain bowls.

Per Serving (2 tablespoons)
calories: 41 | fat: 3.6g
protein: 1.0g | carbs: 1.9g
fiber: 1.1g | sodium: 148mg

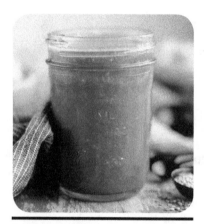

Asian-Inspired Vinaigrette

Prep time: 5 minutes | Cook time: 0 minutes
Serves 2

¼ cup extra-virgin olive oil
3 tablespoons apple cider vinegar
1 garlic clove, minced
1 tablespoon peeled and grated fresh ginger
1 tablespoon chopped fresh cilantro
1 tablespoon freshly squeezed lime juice
½ teaspoon sriracha

1. Add all the ingredients in a small bowl and stir to mix well.
2. Serve immediately, or store covered in the refrigerator and shake before using.

Tips: You can adjust the spiciness by adjusting the sriracha quantity. If you'd like to raise the heat levels, you can add ½ teaspoon of Chinese hot mustard to the vinaigrette. It can be used as a marinade for poultry, meats, fish or seafood.

Per Serving
calories: 251 | fat: 26.8g
protein: 0g | carbs: 1.8g
fiber: 0.7g | sodium: 3mg

Parsley Vinaigrette

Prep time: 5 minutes | Cook time: 0 minutes
Makes about ½ cup

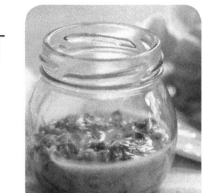

½ cup lightly packed fresh parsley, finely chopped
1/3 cup extra-virgin olive oil
3 tablespoons red wine vinegar
1 garlic clove, minced
¼ teaspoon salt, plus additional as needed

1. Place all the ingredients in a mason jar and cover. Shake vigorously for 1 minute until completely mixed.
2. Taste and add additional salt as needed.
3. Serve immediately or serve chilled.

Tip: If the red wine vinegar isn't available, you can use the apple cider vinegar or rice wine vinegar.

Per Serving (1 tablespoon)
calories: 92 | fat: 10.9g
protein: 0g | carbs: 0g fiber: 0g | sodium: 75mg

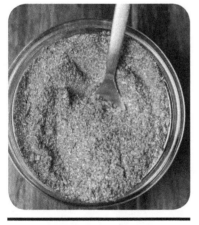

Homemade Blackened Seasoning

Prep time: 10 minutes | Cook time: 0 minutes
Makes about ½ cup

2 tablespoons smoked paprika
2 tablespoons garlic powder
2 tablespoons onion powder
1 tablespoon sweet paprika
1 teaspoon dried dill
1 teaspoon freshly ground black pepper
½ teaspoon ground mustard
¼ teaspoon celery seeds

1. Add all the ingredients to a small bowl and mix well.
2. Serve immediately, or transfer to an airtight container and store in a cool, dry and dark place for up to 3 months.

Tips: You can sprinkle the blackened seasoning on roasted potatoes or broccoli. It also pairs perfectly with blackened codfish or chicken.

Per Serving (1 tablespoon)
calories: 22 | fat: 0.9g
protein: 1.0g | carbs: 4.7g
fiber: 1.0g | sodium: 2mg

Not Old Bay Seasoning

Prep time: 10 minutes | Cook time: 0 minutes
Makes about ½ cup

3 tablespoons sweet paprika
1 tablespoon mustard seeds
2 tablespoons celery seeds
2 teaspoons freshly ground black pepper
1½ teaspoons cayenne pepper
1 teaspoon red pepper flakes
½ teaspoon ground ginger
½ teaspoon ground nutmeg
½ teaspoon ground cinnamon
¼ teaspoon ground cloves

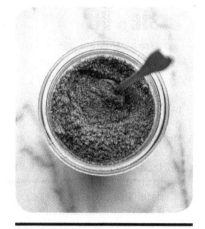

1. Mix together all the ingredients in an airtight container until well combined.
2. You can store it in a cool, dry, and dark place for up to 3 months.

Tip: This seasoning can be used for grilled shrimp, clams, or crab.

Per Serving (1 tablespoon)
calories: 26 | fat: 1.9g
protein: 1.1g | carbs: 3.6g
fiber: 2.1g | sodium: 3mg

Appendix 1: Measurement Conversion Chart

VOLUME EQUIVALENTS(DRY)

US STANDARD	METRIC (APPROXIMATE)
1/8 teaspoon	0.5 mL
1/4 teaspoon	1 mL
1/2 teaspoon	2 mL
3/4 teaspoon	4 mL
1 teaspoon	5 mL
1 tablespoon	15 mL
1/4 cup	59 mL
1/2 cup	118 mL
3/4 cup	177 mL
1 cup	235 mL
2 cups	475 mL
3 cups	700 mL
4 cups	1 L

VOLUME EQUIVALENTS(LIQUID)

US STANDARD	US STANDARD (OUNCES)	METRIC (APPROXIMATE)
2 tablespoons	1 fl.oz.	30 mL
1/4 cup	2 fl.oz.	60 mL
1/2 cup	4 fl.oz.	120 mL
1 cup	8 fl.oz.	240 mL
1 1/2 cup	12 fl.oz.	355 mL
2 cups or 1 pint	16 fl.oz.	475 mL
4 cups or 1 quart	32 fl.oz.	1 L
1 gallon	128 fl.oz.	4 L

TEMPERATURES EQUIVALENTS

FAHRENHEIT(F)	CELSIUS(C) (APPROXIMATE)
225 °F	107 °C
250 °F	120 °C
275 °F	135 °C
300 °F	150 °C
325 °F	160 °C
350 °F	180 °C
375 °F	190 °C
400 °F	205 °C
425 °F	220 °C
450 °F	235 °C
475 °F	245 °C
500 °F	260 °C

WEIGHT EQUIVALENTS

US STANDARD	METRIC (APPROXIMATE)
1 ounce	28 g
2 ounces	57 g
5 ounces	142 g
10 ounces	284 g
15 ounces	425 g
16 ounces (1 pound)	455 g
1.5 pounds	680 g
2 pounds	907 g

Appendix 2: Recipes Index